VINEGAR

250 PRACTICAL USES IN THE HOME

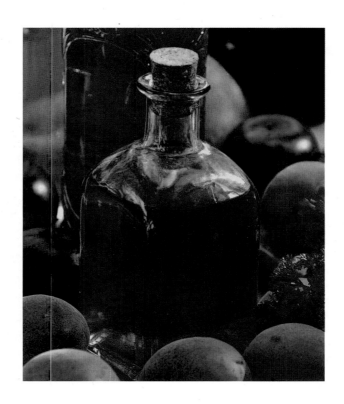

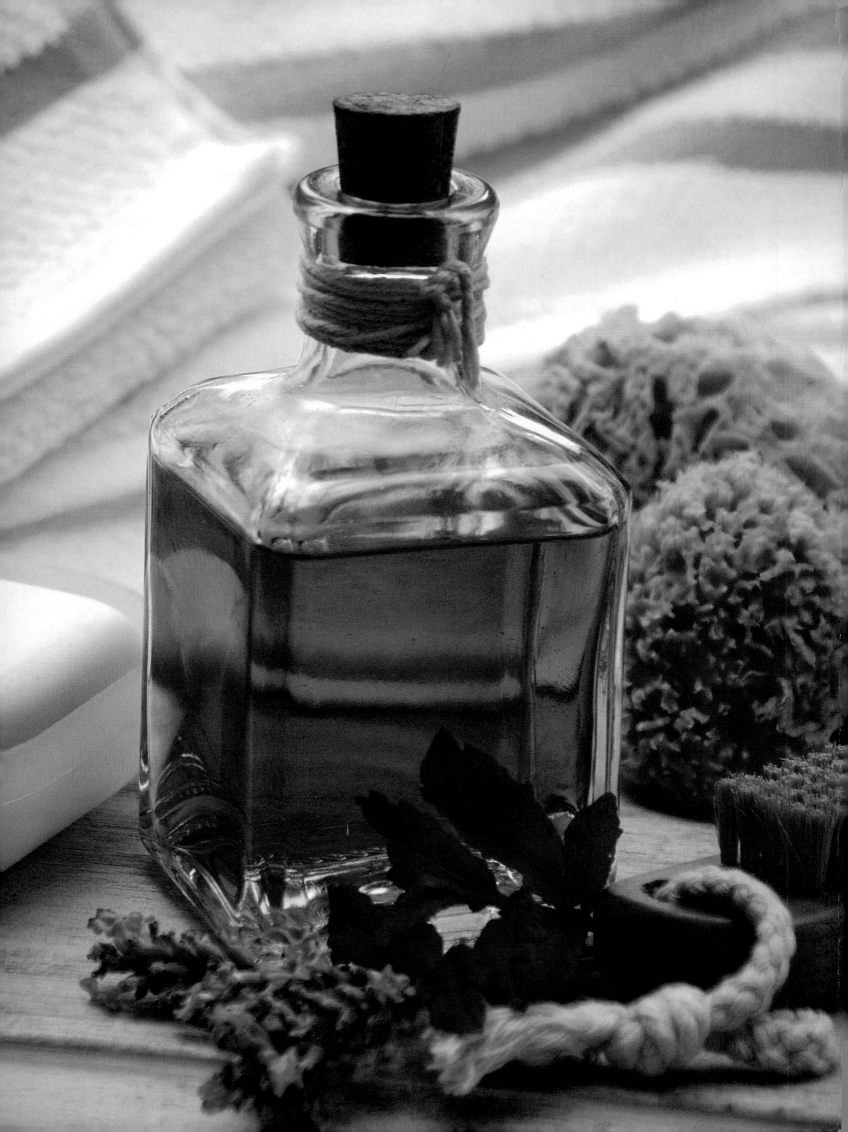

VINEGAR

250 PRACTICAL USES IN THE HOME

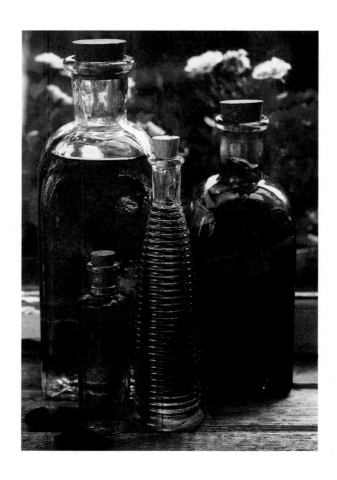

HEALTH • HEALING • BEAUTY • HOMECARE • COOKING

BRIDGET JONES

southwater

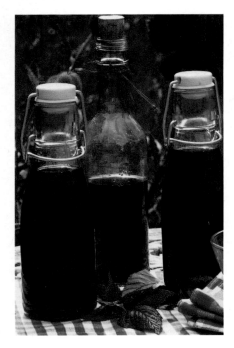

This edition is published by Southwater, an imprint of Anness Publishing Ltd, Blaby Road, Wigston, Leicestershire LE18 4SE

Email: info@anness.com

Web: www.southwaterbooks.com; www.annesspublishing.com

If you like the images in this book and would like to investigate using them for publishing, promotions or advertising, please visit our website www.practicalpictures.com for more information.

Publisher: Joanna Lorenz
Editorial Director: Helen Sudell
Executive Editor: Joanne Rippin
Project Editor: Amy Christian
Photography and styling: Michelle Garrett
Additional photography (recipes): Frank Adam, Edward Allwright, David Armstrong, Tim Auty, Steve Baxter, Martin Brigdale, Nicki Dowey, James Duncan, Gus Filgate, Will Heap, Amanda Heywood, Ferguson Hill, Janine Hosegood, David Jordan, David King, William Lingwood, Patrick McLeavey, Thomas Odulate, Craig Robertson, Gareth Sambridge, Sam Smith, Sam Stowell, Jon Whitaker.
Designer: Sarah Rock
Jacket Design: Adelle Morris
Production Controller: Bessie Bai

ETHICAL TRADING POLICY

At Anness Publishing we believe that business should be conducted in an ethical and ecologically sustainable way, with respect for the environment and a proper regard to the replacement of the natural resources we employ.

As a publisher, we use a lot of wood pulp in high-quality paper for printing, and that wood commonly comes from spruce trees. We are therefore currently growing more than 750,000 trees in three Scottish forest plantations: Berrymoss (130 hectares/320 acres), West Touxhill (125 hectares/305 acres) and Deveron Forest (75 hectares/185 acres). The forests we manage contain more than 3.5 times the number of trees employed each year in making paper for the books we manufacture.

Because of this ongoing ecological investment programme, you, as our customer, can have the pleasure and reassurance of knowing that a tree is being cultivated on your behalf to naturally replace the materials used to make the book you are holding.

Our forestry programme is run in accordance with the UK Woodland Assurance Scheme (UKWAS) and will be certified by the internationally recognized Forest Stewardship Council (FSC). The FSC is a non-government organization dedicated to promoting responsible management of the world's forests. Certification ensures forests are managed in an environmentally sustainable and socially responsible way. For further information about this scheme, go to www.annesspublishing.com/trees

Previously published as part of a larger volume; *Vinegar and Oil*

PUBLISHER'S NOTE

Although the advice and information in this book are believed to be accurate and true at the time of going to press, neither the authors nor the publisher can accept any legal responsibility or liability for any errors or omissions that may have been made nor for any inaccuracies nor for any loss, harm or injury that comes about from following instructions or advice in this book.

NOTES

Bracketed terms are intended for American readers. For all recipes, quantities are given in both metric and imperial measures and, where appropriate, in standard cups and spoons. Follow one set of measures, but not a mixture, because they are not interchangeable.

Standard spoon and cup measures are level. 1 tsp = 5ml, 1 tbsp = 15ml, 1 cup = 250ml/8fl oz.

Australian standard tablespoons are 20ml. Australian readers should use 3 tsp in place of 1 tbsp for measuring small quantities.

American pints are 16fl oz/2 cups. American readers should use 20fl oz/2.5 cups in place of 1 pint when measuring liquids.

Electric oven temperatures in this book are for conventional ovens. When using a fan oven, the temperature will probably need to be reduced by about 10–20°C/20–40°F. Since ovens vary, you should check with your manufacturer's instruction book for guidance. Medium (US large) eggs are used unless otherwise stated.

The nutritional analysis given for each recipe is calculated per portion (i.e. serving or item), unless otherwise stated. If the recipe gives a range, such as Serves 4–6, then the nutritional analysis will be for the smaller portion size, i.e. 6 servings. The analysis does not include optional ingredients, such as salt added to taste.

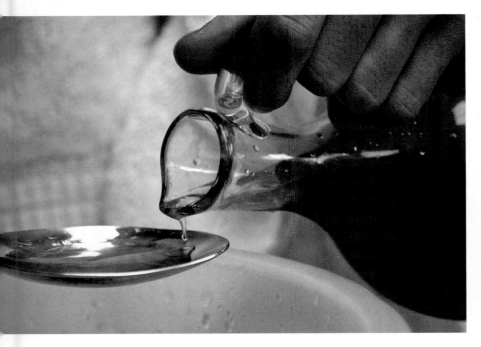

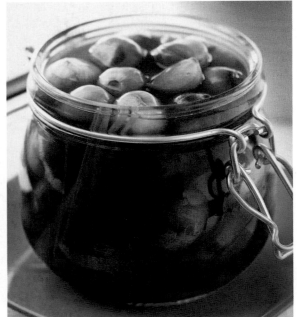

CONTENTS

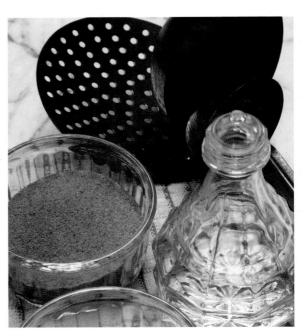

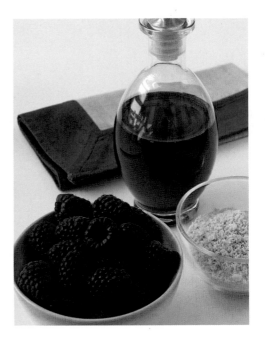

INTRODUCTION

We are all familiar with the basic culinary uses of vinegar, but this book sets out to explore the great all-round potential of this everyday ingredient.

The far-reaching benefits of this ancient ingredient have been recognized in many different cultures throughout the ages. Although nowadays it is most often put to use in the kitchen, vinegar can be applied to a huge variety of tasks.

The properties of vinegar
Vinegar is an astringent, or type of antiseptic, with the ability to clean and remove impurities. Its acidic characteristic also makes vinegar the primary long-term food preservative, used to prevent the growth of bacteria and deterioration. The sharpness of vinegar has the capacity to spotlight flavours, accentuating them and bringing out distinct contrasts.

Culinary essential
Steeped in history but still vital today, vinegar has survived advances in food technology and is still used to preserve many everyday food items, just as it was 2000 years ago. It is also the main ingredient in condiments and bottled sauces, dressings and relishes, with an essential role in the domestic kitchen as well in the food industry.

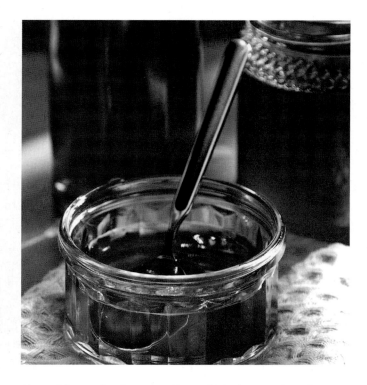

Above: Vinegar has been used in cooking since ancient times.

Utility value
Instead of harsh chemicals and the unwanted films and residues from cans of spray-and-wipe solutions, these natural substances are ideal for restoring fine furniture and for helping to keep the home clean, fresh and eco-friendly.

In the garden vinegar can provide quick, easy and environmentally friendly solutions for many simple problems. From pest control to mould removal, vinegar is increasingly appreciated, and as a natural, non-toxic substance, it is safe to use around children or pets.

Health and beauty
Vinegar has a long-standing reputation for promoting good health and enhancing beauty. It has been used in first aid and providing long-term benefits to the health of skin, hair and nails. Previous generations have made the most of the amazing properties of vinegar, along with other natural ingredients, to complement commercial beauty products and medicines. Simple preparations can still be made at home for a fraction of the price of expensive, branded products. With a growing awareness of the need to respect our environment and an increased emphasis on the importance of including simple unprocessed products in our health and beauty regimes, this is more relevant today than ever before.

Exciting potential
The chapters in this book offer a glimpse of the ancient origins of vinegar, showing the fascinating ways it has been put to use over the centuries. A detailed directory outlines the many different types of vinegar, and practical chapters show the ways it can be used for health and healing, for natural beauty, around the home and in the garden. The book ends with an inspiring selection of tips and recipes for using this essential astringent in the kitchen. Rediscovering the many efficacious uses for vinegar and trying some of the remedies, potions and lotions that our grandparents used, or remember, is great fun, and gives great results with very little expense.

Right: Vinegar has long been an essential culinary ingredient, and is used in the preservation of many foods.

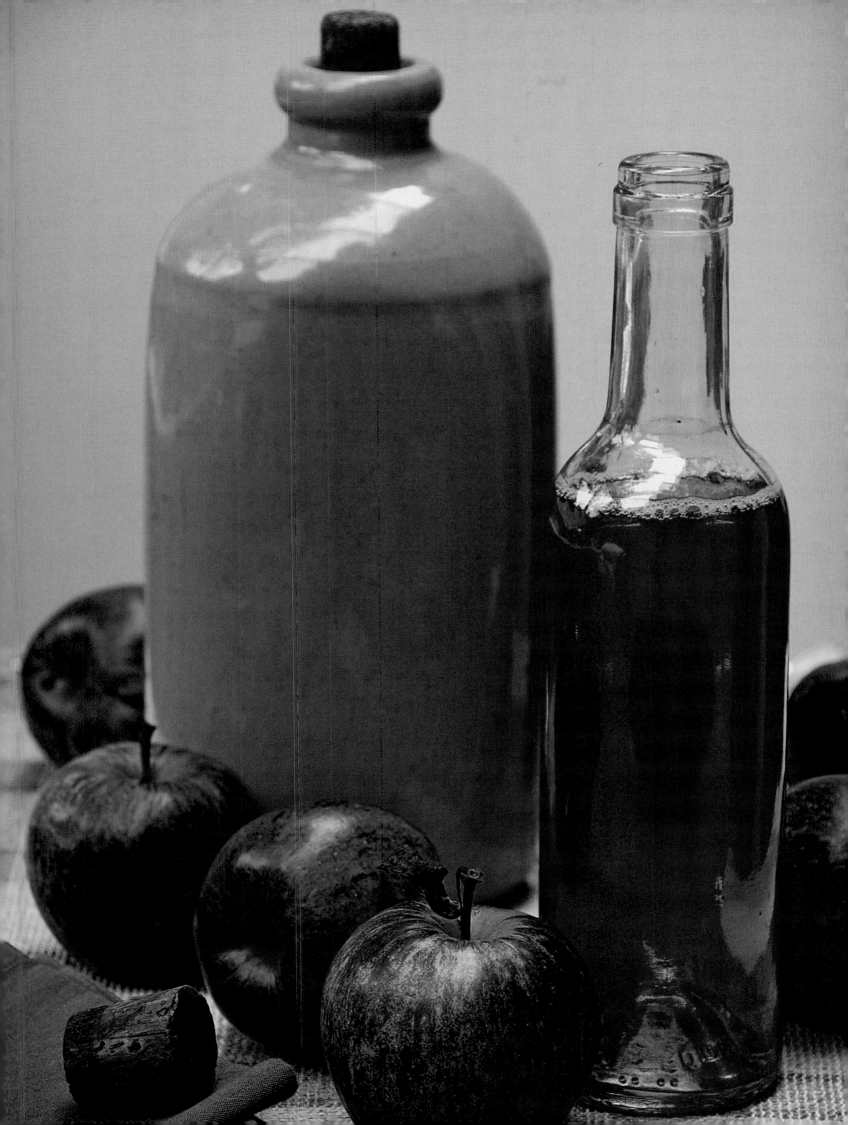

VINEGAR IN HISTORY

Vinegar is an ancient and global ingredient that has been utilized by human beings for so long that its exact origins, or discovery, cannot be traced precisely.

Vinegar is an acid produced when certain bacteria attack alcohol. The first experiences of vinegar were unwelcome accidents of nature. In ancient times, when wine turned sour, the resulting liquor, an unwanted by-product of wine making, was seen as a disaster rather than a triumph.

The useful properties of the soured wine, or vinegar, as a preservative were probably first discovered by chance some 10,000 years ago. It was later, around 5000BC, that the Babylonians began to produce vinegar intentionally and put it to practical use both as a preservative and for culinary purposes. They discovered that the soured wine could be flavoured for use as a condiment. From their wines made from date palm, they produced vinegar infused with herbs and spices.

Egyptian archaeologists have unearthed vessels from around 3000BC believed to have stored vinegar.

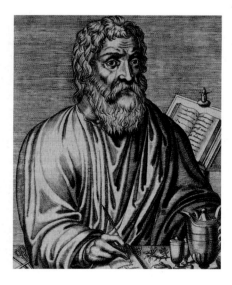

Above: Hippocrates prescribed vinegar and honey to his patients to balance the 'humours' in the body.

Evidence for Greek and Roman use of vinegar as a condiment includes the remains of bowls, called oxybaphon and acetabulum, that were used for serving vinegar at the table so that bread could be dipped into it. The early use of vinegar for moistening bread continued through Biblical times.

Vinegar and the Bible

There are many Biblical references to vinegar, but the most famous must be to a sponge soaked in wine vinegar offered to Jesus as he was dying on the cross: 'When Jesus therefore had received the vinegar, he said, "It is finished." He bowed his head, and gave up his spirit.' (John 19:30) Generally interpreted as an act of mockery, other mentions of vinegar indicated that it may have been an act of kindness. Vinegar was believed to draw out every last bit of moisture from the skin in the mouth to provide some brief comfort in swallowing, and it was also believed to have restorative qualities.

Among earlier Old Testament references to wine vinegar as a drink, there was an instruction to Moses to forbid the Israelites from drinking vinegar made from wine (as well as any other fermented drink). For her work harvesting barley, Ruth was offered bread to dip in wine vinegar, a sign of friendship and acceptance.

One of the Proverbs of Solomon that warned against employing the lazy (sluggards) indicated that vinegar was probably widely consumed and that drinking too much was known

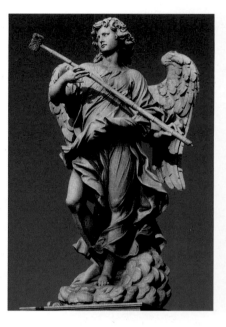

Above: An angel holds a vinegar-soaked sponge, representing the vinegar offered to Jesus on the cross.

not to be good for the teeth. Another proverb implied that the reaction of vinegar mixed with nitre, a name for sodium carbonate or washing soda, was widely understood.

Hippocrates and health

Before Biblical references to vinegar as a restorative drink, it had been widely regarded as a valuable aid to health by the Egyptians, Greeks and Romans. The health benefits of vinegar were acknowledged by Hippocrates, the Greek physician (460–370BC). Often referred to as the father of modern medicine, Hippocrates documented the importance of hygiene and based his theories on the need to achieve a balance for good health. The balance he referred to was with reference to

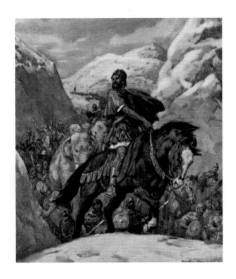

Above: Hannibal used vinegar to break down rocks as he crossed the Alps.

the 'humours' of the body, thought to be blood, phlegm, yellow and black bile. He prescribed both cider vinegar and honey, together and separately, as a balancing tonic to help cure many ailments.

During the 14th to 18th centuries when the plague was evident throughout Europe, vinegar was used as an antiseptic and rubbed into the skin in an effort to avoid infection. The disease was so virulent in 18th-century France that prisoners, who were considered to be expendable, were released to bury the dead. A group of thieves who stole from the corpses they buried survived by cleaning themselves with vinegar to avoid infection and by drinking vinegar infused with garlic, a natural antiseptic. Garlic vinegar is still sometimes referred to as 'four thieves vinegar' for its legendary protective powers against the plague.

Vinegar was used as a deodorizer as well as an antiseptic. When the gentry and ladies of the 17th and 18th centuries walked out on streets that reeked of sewage and waste, they masked their mouths and noses with sponges soaked in vinegar to protect themselves against both the odours of the common people and the potential for contamination.

Small silver boxes and compartments in the tops of walking sticks were designed to hold the little vinegar-soaked sponges.

Military use of vinegar

From ancient to modern times, and worldwide, vinegar was used to promote good health among military ranks. Roman soldiers consumed vinegar to promote good health. They combined vinegar with honey and diluted it to make drinks.

Around 218BC the Carthaginian general Hannibal's army was said to have used vinegar to assist in breaking up rock when clearing a way through the Alps in the advance on Italy. Fires were lit to heat impenetrable rocks, which were then soaked with vinegar. The heating and soaking in acid softened the rock enough to allow the soldiers to break them down into boulders that could be cleared away.

In the 17th century, Louis XIII of France was said to have paid handsomely for vinegar to cool and clean the cannons used in battle. Cleaning the metal with vinegar helped to prevent rusting as well as removing dirt.

During the American Civil War (1861–5) apple cider vinegar was consumed by soldiers to treat scurvy, and as late as the beginning of the 20th century, across the Atlantic, soldiers in the First World War resorted to using vinegar as an antiseptic for those wounded in battle.

Clever Cleopatra

Hannibal was not the only leader to use the powers of vinegar for dissolving solid objects. The Egyptian queen Cleopatra (68–30BC) used vinegar for a more frivolous purpose, to dissolve a pearl. She drank the resulting liquid as a clever way of winning a bet about consuming the most expensive meal by literally consuming the huge cost of the pearl.

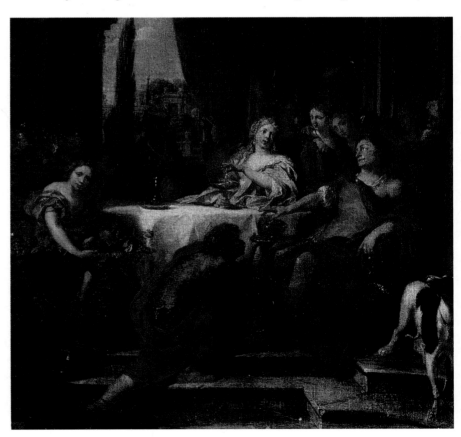

Above: Cleopatra won a bet with Mark Antony by dissolving a pearl in wine vinegar.

THE ENDURANCE OF VINEGAR

Production methods may have progressed, and many varieties of vinegar developed, but the basic uses for vinegar have remained the same through the ages.

Vinegar is a product with a well-founded history as an essential ingredient and basic household item. Different vinegars have maintained their roles for thousands of years, whether for cleaning, health, beauty, cooking or preservation. Vinegar is a product which has to be made, rather than occurring naturally, but efforts put into producing vinegar have long been rewarded by its usefulness.

European cottage industries
The ancient Greeks, Romans and Egyptians set up the first formal vinegar production and storage systems, but following the decline of the Roman Empire, wine (and therefore vinegar) production decreased. Wine and beer were produced on a small scale and so when the value of vinegar as a culinary and household treasure was rediscovered in medieval Europe, its production was very much a cottage industry. Vinegar was a by-product of the alcohol production process, and was made in home breweries and small vineyards, rather than in large specialist vinegar factories.

In Paris, vinegar made from the produce of local vineyards was sold by street vendors, who would roll barrels or carts from door to door. The vendors hailed housekeepers and persuaded them of the quality of their 'vinaigre'. It was during the 14th century that a commercial vinegar production corporation was set up in Paris.

In Great Britain the production of malt vinegar, or 'alegar', was so profitable that a vinegar tax was established in 1673 by an Act of Parliament.

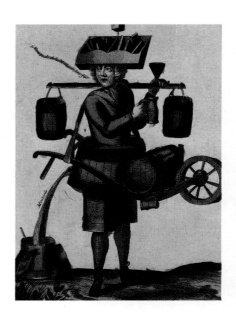

Above: This 17th-century engraving shows a French vinegar seller.

Development of Italian vinegars
The town of Modena in Italy had also been producing and maturing vinegar since the Middle Ages. Records indicate that the sweet vinegar syrup of Modena was sold from the 14th century. By the 17th century fashionable households boasted their own stores of 'balsamico', a product that had developed an amazing reputation. It was even said to be capable of bringing the dead back to life. Modena remains the centre for balsamic vinegar production today (along with nearby Reggio Emilia). The name 'Aceto Balsamico Tradizionale di Modena' is protected by the European Union's Protected Designation of Origin (PDO).

Cider vinegar in the United States
Introduced by early European settlers, apples were used in the United States for eating, cooking, and to feed livestock.

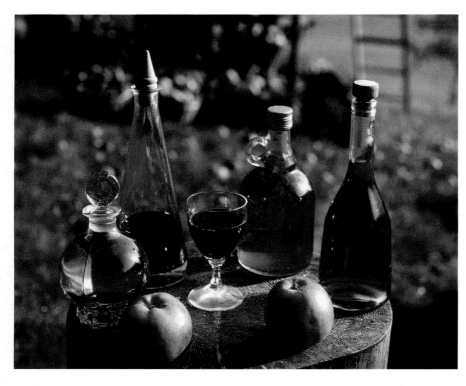

Above: Cider vinegar has been the most popular vinegar in the US since the 18th century.

Apples were also pressed to make apple juice, a portion of which was fermented into cider, allowing it to be stored over the winter months. Some of the cider was allowed to ferment further into cider vinegar, which was prized for its many uses – as a medicine, a condiment, a preserving liquid, for cleaning and a host of other household duties.

During the 18th and 19th centuries, American farm labourers would consume 'switchel', a drink made from cider vinegar mixed with water and ginger and sweetened with honey. Switchel served as an early energy drink for the exhausted workers out in the field. By the early 1800s cider vinegar was selling for three times the price of apple cider.

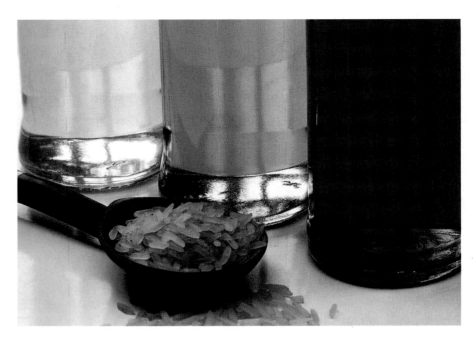

Above: Vinegars made from different ingredients are found all over the world. Vinegar made from rice was used in ancient Chinese medicine as well as in cooking.

Chinese and Japanese vinegars

Vinegar has always featured in oriental medicines and diets. Although much of the history of the discovery of vinegar and development of commercial production focuses on the wine and malt vinegar industries, rice has been used for producing vinegar in both Japan and China since ancient times (Chinese records dating back to 1200BC include references to vinegar). Rice vinegar is still a vital cooking ingredient in these countries and is used in Chinese medicine.

Value of vinegar now

The fundamental uses of vinegar have stayed much the same for several hundred years, with increased interest in the role that vinegar can play to promote health and well-being. Even though there are now many expensive vinegars available, standard vinegar still has a high profile in the supermarket and a place in home store cupboards.

Everyday chores As the array of harsh household cleaners and chemicals has expanded, it is good to find a simple

yet effective alternative that is easy to use and inexpensive. Vinegar is a practical choice for use as an everyday home-cleaning product as well as for renovating and deep cleaning.

Natural balance At the same time as trying to minimize household use of potentially harmful products, many people are also looking for natural ways of building up resistance to illness and infection, and of averting or counteracting relatively minor conditions. Instead of dashing to the pharmacy for every little complaint, there is a growing trend to use simple cures for minor irritations.

Simple skin care Legend has it that Helen of Troy (described as the most beautiful woman ever in Greek mythology) bathed in vinegar. While this may be a little extreme, vinegar has been used for centuries for refreshing baths, face and hair washes and it is still popular. Alternatives are increasingly being sought to replace high-tech beauty products. Simple, inexpensive blends are welcomed by those who would prefer to minimize their use of complicated and often expensive beauty ranges.

Gourmet ingredient The history of vinegar suggests that it was originally most valued for its health-giving properties. It was used in even greater quantities than it is now as a restoring and refreshing drink, and to aid digestion.

Vinegar has been used in preservation throughout history, for pickling fish and meat as well as fruit and vegetables. It plays a vital role in the preparation of classic French sauces and in the sweet-sour or hot-sour flavours of Chinese cooking.

An increase in the availability of different types of vinegar has led to a growing appreciation of the sometimes subtle distinctions in flavour between the many varieties. In recent decades, vinegar has become more than a tonic, vital culinary acid or simple souring agent, and has become increasingly seen as a gourmet ingredient. There are many that are used with discretion for their flavour nuances. Vinegar has developed from a basic store-cupboard ingredient to a highly-prized condiment, of which there are now many types to choose from.

FROM ALCOHOL TO VINEGAR

In essence, vinegar is the product of a natural process of fermentation, for example, of fruit, barley or rice, followed by bacterial activity.

The basic ingredients of vinegar, such as grapes, other fruit, malted barley or rice, are fermented to produce alcohol and then a bacteria culture is added to produce the acidic vinegar. The flavour of the original ingredients is often retained and, being acidic, the vinegar tastes sharp. The combination of sharpness and flavour nuances gives vinegar its culinary value.

Fermentation

The first step towards vinegar being made is a process called alcoholic fermentation. The process happens in nature, for example when yeasts react with the natural sugar (glucose) and water in ripening fruit to produce alcohol in the form of ethanol.

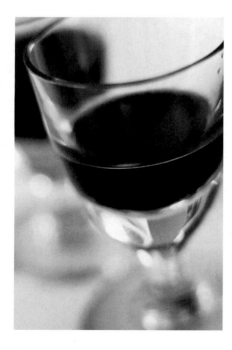

Above: Vinegar is formed when bacteria in fermenting alcohol produce acetic acid.

To complete the chemical equation, carbon dioxide (CO_2) and heat are given off as by-products of the reaction. Compounds called esters also develop during the reaction, producing fruit flavours in the vinegar.

The commercial fermentation process is a controlled version of what happens in nature. Wild yeasts do not necessarily produce pleasing flavours, so specific strains of yeast are used for making wines and beers. By controlling the yeasts and the process, the fruit base (or grain in the case of beer) is fermented under controlled conditions to produce alcohol with a good flavour. When all the sugar has been used the process will stop, because the yeast needs food in order to live and multiply. Alternatively, when the alcohol level becomes too high, the yeasts will not survive.

From alcohol to acid

Anyone who has tried wine-making or brewing their own beer at home will know that the sugar concentration and temperature, along with cleanliness, are very important. Equipment has to be sterilized and air must be excluded from the fermenting liquid for any chance of success, otherwise the wine or beer can develop very unpleasant off-flavours. In the same way that yeasts are present in nature, some bacteria naturally present in fruit or carried in the air will work on the alcohol and break it down into acid.

MOTHER OF VINEGAR

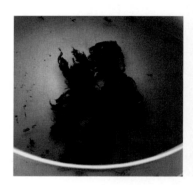

It is vital to preserve the particular strains of aerobic bacteria, or *acetobacter aceti*, which are used to ferment the wine or other base and which produce acetic acid along with good flavour.

In the traditional production methods, the bacteria form a slimy, slightly cloudy string or surface on the fermenting vinegar and this is known as the mother of vinegar, vinegar mother, or simply the mother. The mother of vinegar forms on the surface because there it has access to air.

In classic techniques, enough mother of vinegar is retained to continue the vinegar-making process. Before pasteurization was a standard process used for inexpensive vinegar, a half-empty bottle of vinegar stored in a warm place, or in direct sunlight, would soon develop a mother of vinegar which could clearly be seen floating in the liquid.

The bacteria need a supply of oxygen to produce acetic acid from the ethanol, so there has to be air in the brewing container. Fermenting beer or wine left open to air, perhaps in equipment that was not properly cleaned after previous use, is likely to become acidic and more like vinegar, which is a disaster for the home wine maker or brewer who anticipated sipping a successful liquor but found that they were left with sharp-tasting vinegar instead.

From acid to vinegar

In commercial vinegar production, the bacteria *acetobacter aceti* are desirable, and are deliberately added to the fermented alcohol. When there is oxygen present, the bacteria will turn the alcohol into acetic acid, which is one of the main components of vinegar.

Many centuries ago the first vinegar was made by the accidental presence of bacteria in fermenting alcohol. Once vinegar was valued in its own right, the process was encouraged and vinegar was eventually put to positive use as a preservative. Over the generations, vinegar has grown from being a by-product of wine, beer or other alcohol, and a large specialist vinegar industry has developed.

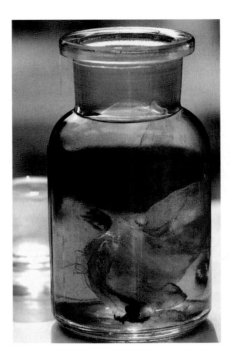

Above: If a bottle of unpasteurized vinegar is left opened, the presence of oxygen means that a mother will soon develop.

Vinegar producers take a great deal of care to select beer or wine of the best quality for their vinegar and to ensure that the conditions are exactly right for avoiding contamination by any unwanted bacteria that might produce any undesirable off-flavours in the vinegar.

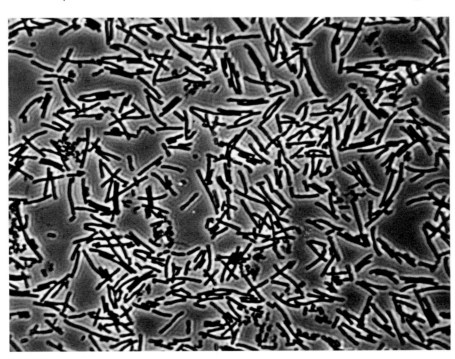

Above: The acetobacter aceti *bacteria which produce acetic acid from alcohol.*

ACETIC ACID

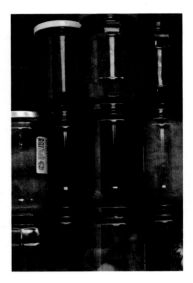

Acetic acid, which is also known as ethanoic acid, is the main ingredient (besides water) in vinegar, and gives it its sour taste. It is important to differentiate however between vinegar made from a traditional ingredient base and diluted acetic acid which is made from ethanol and has none of the positive qualities of vinegar.

Vinegar is made from a base ingredient such as barley, fruit or rice. The naturally occurring yeasts in these ingredients react with sugar and produce compounds called esters that contribute the flavour to the vinegar. Instead of a food base, industrial acetic acid can be produced from ethanol (pure alcohol).

Acetic acid is very sharp and often used in preserves and pickles instead of vinegar. It may be useful as a preservative but it contributes no flavour and makes the food taste particularly bitter; even sweetened pickles made with acetic acid have an unmistakable harshness. The best advice is always to carefully check the labels on pickles and other products that would traditionally use vinegar (such as salad dressings and condiments) because acetic acid may be used instead. It is also a good idea to check out the labels on wine vinegars, particularly the less expensive types that look as though they are full flavoured and matured – they may actually be simple vinegars combined with sweetening and flavouring ingredients.

VINEGAR AS AN ACID

Vinegar is an acidic liquid resulting from the fermentation of alcohol. Its acidity is an important factor for its many household uses.

Knowing a little bit about acids and how they relate to, and react with other substances helps to explain why vinegar is so useful for certain household purposes as well as in cooking.

About acids and alkalis

In chemical terms, pure water is neutral, neither acid nor alkali. Acids and alkalis, known as bases, are measured on a scale measured by pH, which stands for potential hydrogen or power of hydrogen and is related to the concentration of hydrogen ions in the liquid. The scale ranges from 0 to 14, with pure water in the middle with a pH of 7. Acids have a pH below 7, getting more acidic as the pH is lowered, so a strong acid would have a pH of 2 to 0.

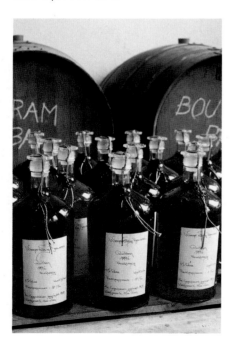

Above: Wine vinegar is created when fermented grapes become acidic.

Alkalis or bases have a pH above 7, with a pH of 12 to 14 being very strong. The scale 0 to 7 is not measured in straightforward increments of 1 but in logarithmic stages. A difference in pH of 1 represents a tenfold difference in strength. Although the difference in figures may seem small, the actual difference in strength of the liquids will be large. A meter is used to test pH.

Properties of acids

Acids can be solids as well as liquids, for example, citric acid is available as crystals as well as in liquid form. Tartaric acid is found in fruit, especially grapes, but a related solid form (or acid salt) of potassium hydrogen tartrate is commonly known as cream of tartar.

Acids have a sharp or sour flavour – citric acid makes citrus fruit taste sharp; the acetic acid in vinegar makes it taste sour. Lactic acid makes some dairy products taste the way they do, for example sour milk, cream or tart soft cheeses have a slightly sharp, tangy or fresh flavour.

Reactions between acids and alkalis

When acids and some alkalis or bases are combined, they react and are neutralized. In the process, another chemical compound or salt is produced and gas given off. This type of chemical reaction can be useful. For example, in baking, mixing cream of tartar (an acid) with bicarbonate of soda (an alkali), adding water and then

TYPICAL pH VALUES

ACID / NEUTRAL / ALKALI	pH	
ACID		strong hydrochloric acid
	pH 1	battery acid
		lemon juice, gastric acid, acetic acid
	pH 3	vinegar, carbonated soft drinks, orange juice, cream of tartar
	pH 4	citric acid, tomato juice, skin, hydrogen peroxide
	pH 5	coffee, handwash liquid
	pH 6	urine, saliva
NEUTRAL	pH 7	distilled water, milk, blood, semen
	pH 8	egg white, bile
	pH 9	bicarbonate of soda (baking soda), borax
	pH 10	washing powder, milk of magnesia
		bleach, laundry ammonia
	pH 12	dishwasher powder, photo developer
	pH 13	lime, lye
ALKALI	pH 14	caustic soda

ACIDS

Vinegar is a mild acetic acid, which is not usually damaging to skin, but strong acids will burn the skin. Strong acids will also attack fabrics (natural and manmade) and cause them to disintegrate.

heating produces a gas, carbon dioxide, that makes the mixture rise. Bubbles of the carbon dioxide are trapped when the mixture bakes. Vinegar, another acid, is used as a raising agent in some baking recipes, when mixed with bicarbonate of soda in the same way. The reaction between acid and alkali is also used in traditional effervescent tablets available for relieving indigestion.

Acids and metals

The reaction between acids and metals can be unwelcome when using cooking equipment, especially uncoated copper, iron or aluminium pans. The flavour of the food can be tainted by the metal and the

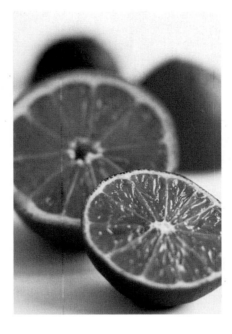

Above: Citrus fruits such as oranges, lemons and limes contain citric acid.

reaction may also produce unwanted toxins. This reaction, although usually seen as a negative one, is however sometimes deliberately used in food preparation. Some old-fashioned cooking equipment was uncoated and this was sometimes valued for the effect it had on the food.

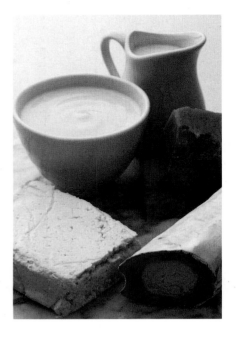

Above: Lactic acid gives some dairy products a sharp, tangy flavour.

For example, when copper preserving pans were used for making jellies and sweet preserves the acid from the fruit reacted with the uncoated copper giving the preserve (if properly prepared) a particularly sparkling clarity, albeit with a small unwanted dose of metal.

Generally, however, the reaction between vinegar (an acid) and metal should be avoided in cooking. When making chutneys and pickles with vinegar as the preservative, care must be taken. When bottling the preserve, uncoated or damaged metal lids should not be used to seal jars or bottles, as the acidic preserve will rapidly corrode the lid, causing damage and ruining the preserve.

The same effect can be found when using aluminium foil as a direct wrapping on food, for example around a rich fruit cake. The acid from the fruit will rapidly corrode the foil, reducing it to a powder. Wrapping the item in baking parchment first prevents the contact and therefore the reaction.

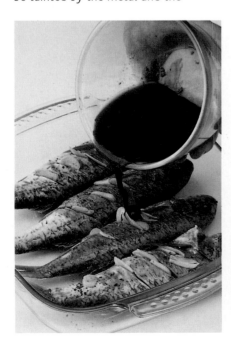

Above: The acidic properties in vinegar make it an excellent base for marinades, used alone or with other ingredients.

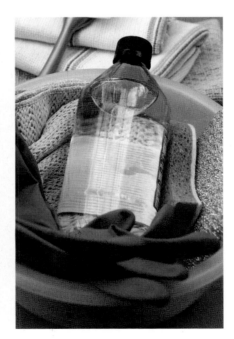

Above: The acetic acid in vinegar allows it to cut through grease and dirt when used as a cleaning agent around the home.

COMMERCIAL VINEGAR PRODUCTION

In vinegar factories, a carefully controlled process guarantees that the fermentation, environment and maturing process produce perfect vinegar.

Methods of production for vinegar ensure that the correct bacteria are used, that the fermentation base is of suitable quality, and the environment for souring allows the required bacteria to work. It is important that foreign fermentations are prevented – these may ruin the flavour of the vinegar. Temperature and exposure to air are standardized along with the length of fermentation. When one batch of vinegar is produced, a small percentage, containing the 'mother', is retained and used to begin the process again. Today there are several different methods used for commercial vinegar production.

The Orléans method

France is famous for refining vinegar production and developing the Orléans method, also known as the continuous method. Orléans, an ancient city of pre-Roman existence on the Loire, was liberated from British rule by Joan of Arc in 1429, by which time it was already famous as a centre for food and wine collection and distribution, as well as for vinegar production. The vinegar industry grew because wines brought to Orléans would often arrive soured in the cask.

King Charles VI officially recognized the vinegar merchants' corporation in 1394. Some 200 years later, just as there were *confréries* or associations, orders or brotherhoods to protect local wine-making standards and traditions, the local profession for vinegar merchants was recognized by King Henri III in 1580.

Local distributors had developed the trade by taking the *vin aigre*, or sour wine, and fermenting it to produce good-quality vinegar rather than letting it go to waste. The process was used only for good-quality wines, which were slowly fermented in the barrel under controlled temperature conditions. Local barrel makers set the standards, ensuring that the barrels were aerated and not over-filled so that the true flavours of the original wine were preserved and carried into the vinegar. Once it had been fermented, the vinegar was also matured.

Vinegar production developed and by the 18th century, Orléans was established as the centre for wine vinegar. The slow and careful process is still used today by specialist vinegar producers and the Orléans method is recognized as a sign of great quality.

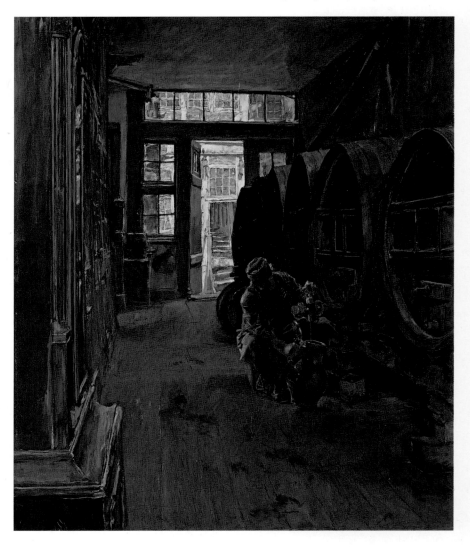

Above: In the Vinegar Factory in Hamburg, *Gotthardt Johann Kuehl, 1891.*

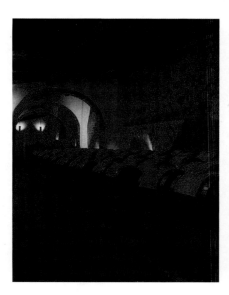

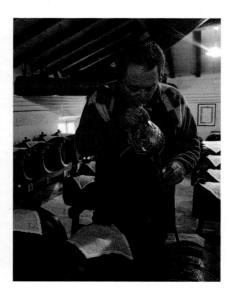

NEMATODE WORMS

These small worms, *turbatrix aceti*, measure about 2mm (1⁄16in) long. When vinegar was produced following traditional techniques, they were very useful – they consume all the debris and dead vinegar bacteria.

They were introduced to the vinegar barrels and would survive for about 10 months, reproducing at a rate of about 45 young for each female.

By performing their vital house-keeping task in the fermentation barrels, the nematode worms helped to prevent any unwanted off-flavours from developing in the vinegar.

Above: Wine vinegars are matured in oak barrels for at least six months.

Above: Balsamic vinegar matures for many years then is tested by skilled producers.

Generator method

The Orléans method of vinegar production is time-consuming. A new generator method, which speeds up the process by fermenting bacteria over a bed of wood shavings, was developed early in the 19th century by a German vinegar producer, Schuezenbach. It is also known as the German or Schuezenbach method as well as the 'quick vinegar' or 'fast acetic' method.

A large surface area of wood shavings (originally beech) was used as the base for the vinegar culture, providing greater exposure to oxygen for the vinegar mother, which reduced the time needed to produce the acetic acid. The liquor was sprayed evenly over the wood shavings. To achieve the required level of acidity, the process could be repeated. Alternatively, the liquor was passed through several aerated barrels or generators over a few days. This was not as efficient as spraying the liquor.

In traditional malt vinegar production, the liquor was trickled down threads on to a bed of beechwood shavings or charcoal that formed the fermentation base. Base ingredients such as beer, brandy, whisky, molasses and honey were used in this way for fermentation and acetic acid production. The disadvantage of using this quicker method was increased evaporation of the alcohol and therefore loss of acetic acid. The quick fermentation generated sufficient heat to destroy some of the natural flavours that would be retained by a cooler, slower process.

Instead of maturing this new vinegar which had been made by the generator or 'quick vinegar' methods, flavouring ingredients, such as caramel (which gave a rich brown colour) were added before the vinegar was sold.

Submerged fermentation method

Further developments soon made vinegar production even quicker. The vinegar mother was submerged in the liquid and air pumped through it for continuous aeration. Temperature and exposure to air were highly controlled and the whole process was sped up to produce a product of reliable basic quality. The disadvantage was that the character or intense flavour found in slow-fermented wine vinegars was lost. This method is used today and produces vinegars for commercial pickling and sauce production.

Finishing fermentation

Once the vinegar has fermented, it is either filtered to remove the mother and debris or may be cleared in a similar way to wine. To prevent unwanted further fermentation, air has to be excluded from the vinegar. Some types of vinegar are pasteurized to kill off the remaining bacteria.

Maturing wine vinegar

The best wine vinegars are matured in barrels that have been used for the purpose for many generations. Skilled vinegar makers ensure that the conditions are right to promote maturation and they assess the quality of their product, checking progress for the point when the wine vinegar has developed yet not lost its fresh acetic quality. While some wine vinegars may need a minimum of six months ageing, the balsamic vinegars of Italy in particular are known for long maturation of up to 50 years or more.

HOME-MADE VINEGAR

Making your own vinegar is fascinating and can be fun, but there are a few pitfalls to avoid and tips to follow for reliable results. Use live – unpasteurized – vinegar as a starting point.

The idea of making vinegar may seem novel now but in the past it was fairly standard practice to keep a vinegar mother on the go for souring wine. Before wine vinegar was readily available, adding the remnants of a bottle of wine to vinegar to ferment down was a good way of making better quality vinegar. It is certainly worth an attempt at making some vinegar – if a decent mother develops, then more adventurous experiments with home-made fruit wines and better-quality vinegar or sherry may be worthwhile.

Traditional methods

The tried and trusted way to make vinegar is to use a barrel with a tap in the bottom and pour in live, organic wine, then add some live (unpasteurized) vinegar that will ferment. The fermentation takes place on the surface of the vinegar, forming a scum of bacteria, the mother. The bacteria need air, so the barrel must not be filled, and it needs to be kept in a warm place. The vinegar can be drawn off through the tap and more wine added. The larger the quantity, the longer the souring will take.

Basic vinegar-making

A simple way of experimenting is to use some wine or cider and live vinegar. Dilute strong wine with water and mix it with some live vinegar. Use a glass or glazed container, not metal or lead crystal – a large jug (pitcher) or crock is ideal for an initial experiment. Cover the jug with muslin (cheesecloth)

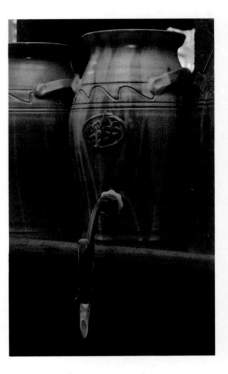

Above: A container with a tap in the bottom is useful when making vinegar.

to allow air in but keep dust and dirt out. Then leave in a warm place, preferably somewhere dark and out of direct sunlight. The temperature should be constant (as for home brewing or wine-making), as off-flavours develop if the fermenting liquid fluctuates between very hot and cold conditions.

The mother of vinegar should form on the surface and this must not be disturbed. Use a drinking straw to remove small samples of the souring wine from the bottom of the jug and check progress over 2–4 weeks. The wine should develop a vinegar-like aroma.

Once the vinegar has reached a strength you are happy with, or if it begins to lose its flavour, it is ready. Once fermented, carefully syphon off

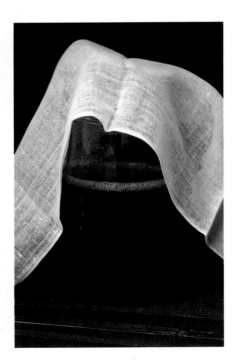

Above: Vinegar can be made easily, at home, in an ordinary jug.

Above: The vinegar needs to be left for between two to four weeks to ferment.

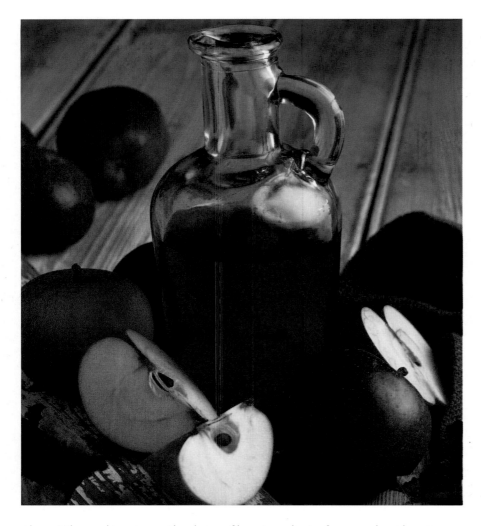

Above: When making vinegar the choice of base ingredient – for example, cider, wine or beer – is important. For a truly do-it-yourself approach, use home-made alcohol.

the vinegar into a separate container, leaving the mother behind with a small amount of vinegar for making the next batch. Strain, place the vinegar in a clean airtight container and store in a cool place to clear. The vinegar should be allowed to mature for at least six months so that the flavour develops. To prevent further unwanted fermentation, Campden tablets (potassium or sodium metabisulphite – available from a brewing supplier) can be added to kill off the bacteria before the vinegar is matured.

Serious home-vinegar production

To produce reliable, good-quality vinegar at home means being more stringent about methods, sterilizing equipment to keep unwanted bacteria from the fermentation and checking both alcohol levels in the wine and acid levels in the vinegar. Home brewing and wine-making suppliers are a good source of equipment, from glazed fermentation crocks and heated mats or jackets designed to maintain constant temperatures for fermentation, to equipment for checking alcohol levels before starting and acid-testing kits. Some suppliers may be able to provide detailed information on making vinegar at home, including supplying suitable starter bacteria. Of course the choice of cider, beer or wine is also important and, with experience, this can be home-made.

TIPS FOR MAKING VINEGAR

- Check out suppliers of the bacteria culture (acetobacter), for example on the Internet or through local wine-making suppliers. Remember, though, that vinegar is anathema to wine makers and some may be affronted by an enquiry about acetobacter; however, many enthusiastic home brewers have experimented with vinegar and are very helpful. If acetobacter is not available, use live organic vinegar as a starter.
- Use organic cider, beer or wine. Alcohol that is chemically treated to prevent further fermentation will not be suitable. For example, potassium sorbate and/or Campden tablets or the equivalent are added to stop micro-organism activity and this will prevent a vinegar mother from forming.
- Check the alcohol content. It should be 5–7 per cent, therefore stronger wines should be diluted with water.
- Acid testing kits (from wine-making suppliers) should be used for checking the acidity level, which should be at least 5 per cent.
- Find somewhere clean and constant in temperature for keeping the culture working. The temperature should be about 16–27°C/60–80°F. Spells of warm weather are ideal, but make sure the temperature does not rise too high during the day or drop sharply at night.
- Sterilize equipment using a solution recommended for baby feeding equipment, rinsing everything thoroughly. Wash the cloth for covering the container in sterilizing fluid.
- The mixture should begin to smell sharp within a few days and take up to a month to become vinegar.
- Strain the vinegar through coffee filter paper when it is sufficiently acidic.
- If the result is good, save some of the vinegar and mother to make another batch.

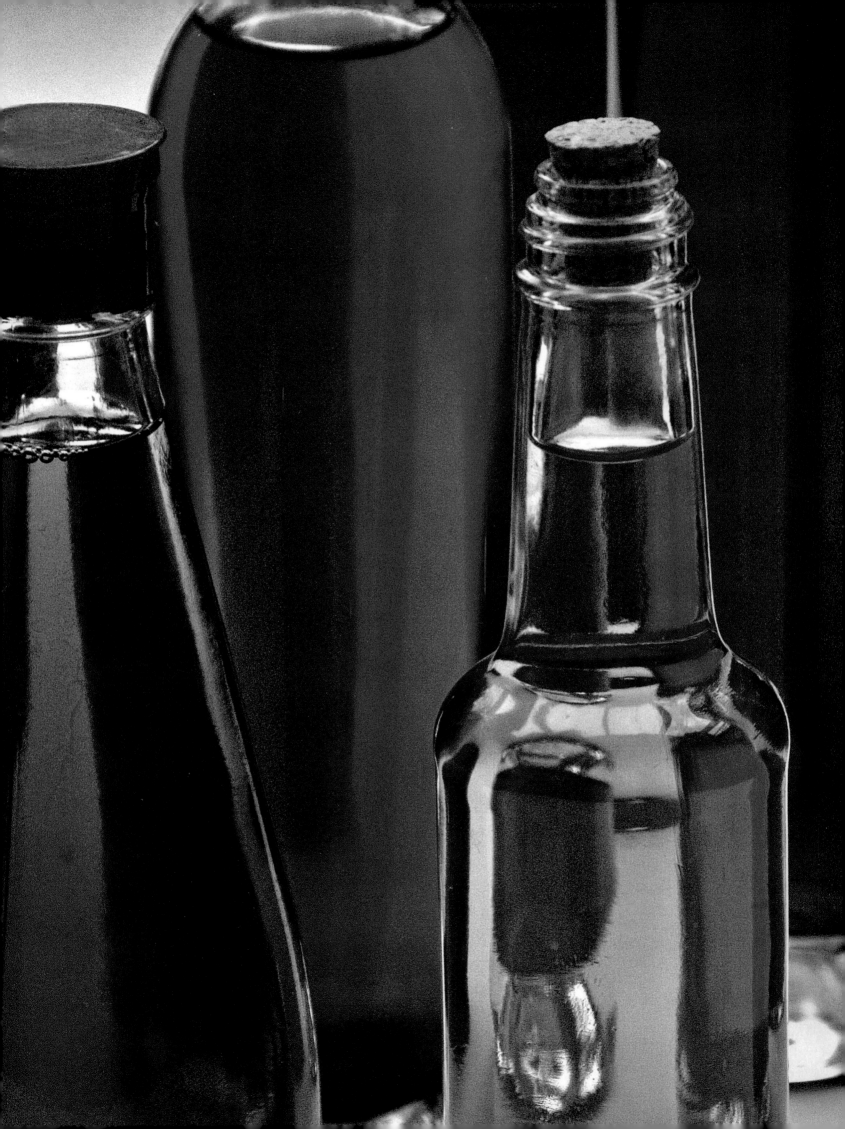

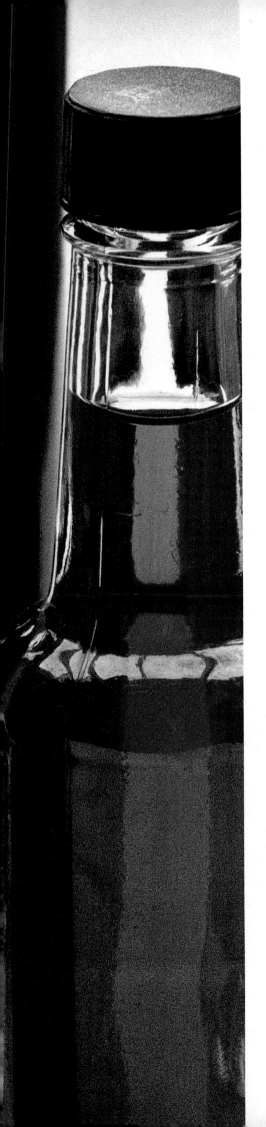

DIRECTORY OF VINEGARS

From crystal-clear distilled malt vinegar to glossy, dark treacle-like balsamic, there is a vinegar to suit each food, every dish and all occasions. Beyond the kitchen, there is a choice of basic vinegars for household use and several types are ideal for simple beauty preparations. All vinegars have some positive contribution to make to health, from antiseptic qualities to promoting good digestion. This section provides a guide to the appearance and properties of all the key types of vinegar.

Left: Vinegars vary in colour and clarity according to the ingredients from which they are made.

A VARIETY OF VINEGARS

Vinegar is an ancient and global ingredient, so it is not surprising that there is now an amazing selection from which to choose. Different vinegars suit different purposes, so choose with care.

The first discovery of vinegar was in soured wine, but since then many different varieties of vinegar have been manufactured. Ale was also traditionally used for producing 'alegar' or sour ale. Beer, ale, cider, mead, sherry or perry (fermented from pears) can all be used as a base for vinegar, or fruit juices or mashes may be the starting point for fermenting through alcohol to acetic acid. Besides grapes or apples, raspberries and other berries, or dates, figs and stone (pit) fruit are traditionally used to make vinegar. Dried fruit, as well as fresh, can be fermented into vinegar. Sugar cane, molasses and glucose or corn syrup are also used.

Rice is the base for many Chinese and Japanese vinegars but other grains, such as millet and barley, can be used. Cherries, peaches, dates, grapes and honey have all played a part in Chinese vinegar-making history. Other South-east Asian vinegars are made from coconut water and palm sap.

One of the most unusual base ingredients must be whey, the liquid left after producing cheese curds, which was fermented by a Swiss vinegar producer early in the 20th century. It is unlikely to feature on the average supermarket shelf, but whey vinegar is still available as a healthfood product.

Choosing vinegars

The type of vinegar should not be seen as a guide to quality but of taste and style, and suitability for different uses. Quality depends on the basic ingredients used, the fermentation process and whether or not the vinegar has been matured. Select vinegars to suit different culinary purposes or other needs; for example, a malt vinegar may be suitable for certain pickles while wine vinegar may be ideal for simple dressings to coat everyday mixed salads. Superior wine vinegar may be reserved for dressing individual fruit or vegetables, to deglaze cooking pans or for adding piquancy to sweet dishes.

The best advice is to experiment with different types and brands, buying small quantities that can be used up relatively quickly.

Most large supermarkets offer a wide variety of vinegars but it is also worth remembering that wine merchants sometimes sell vinegars from small producers. Delicatessens, organic shops and markets, wholefood shops and speciality food stores are all great places to discover vinegars from around the world.

Organic vinegars

Vinegars produced to organic standards are widely available, especially cider vinegars. Some unpasteurized organic vinegars may contain live bacteria that could develop a mother of vinegar once the contents of the bottle are part used, exposing the surface of the

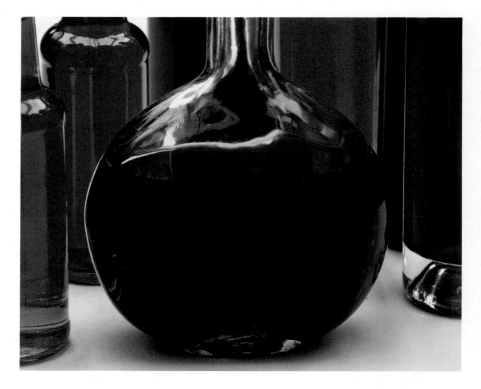

Above: Different vinegars have been produced all over the world for centuries. The ingredients and method of production influence the overall quality of each vinegar.

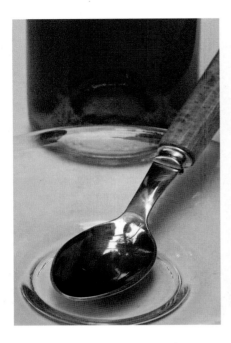

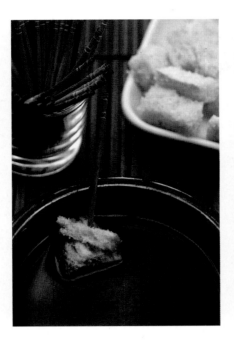

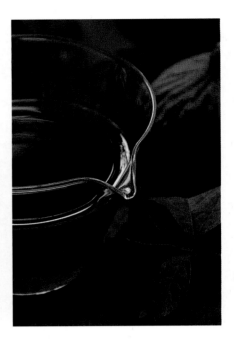

Above: Taste one or two types of vinegar by sipping a small amount from a spoon.

Above: Dip small cubes of white bread into vinegar to compare several types.

Above: Vinegar can be made from different fruit or vegetables.

vinegar to air. This could be useful for anyone wanting to try making their own vinegar.

Tasting tips

Take advantage of vinegar tasting sessions offered by wine merchants, supermarkets or other specialist stores. It is a very good way of sampling and comparing different brands and qualities of the same type of vinegar.

It is also worthwhile comparing a couple of different vinegars at home. Sipping a little off a teaspoon is the obvious way of tasting, drinking plain water between samples, but it is better to dip small cubes of good-quality, close-textured white bread into a small amount of vinegar. Make the cubes similar in size and without crust. Pour a little vinegar on a saucer and lightly dip the bread in it. This is a good way of comparing the sharpness and additional flavours in different vinegars. Drink water between samples and compare only two or three types at once to avoid confusion.

Make a note of impressions on a label, with ideas for using the vinegar, then tie it around the bottle. Experiment with the suggestion soon afterwards to confirm or correct the first impression.

Alternative ingredients

While the majority of commercial vinegars are based on wine, ale or a fermented fruit or grain base, all sorts of different ingredients are used for small-scale production. These vinegars are not generally available in the average supermarket but independent delicatessens, wholefood or healthfood stores and mail order specialist suppliers are the best places to find and sample the more unusual end of the vinegar spectrum.

Millet, wheat, sorghum and oats may all be used in the same way as rice or barley. The sap of palm trees is also used in vinegars, particularly in the Philippines. A wide variety of vegetables, including potatoes, beetroot (beet), carrot, asparagus and cucumbers are also used for making specialist brewed vinegars.

STORING VINEGAR

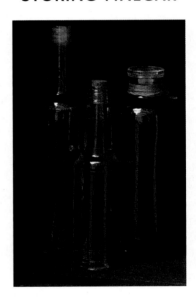

All varieties of vinegar should be stored in an airtight bottle in a cool, dark place. Those vinegars with live bacteria remaining will begin to ferment if they are not stored in this way.

Pasteurized or distilled vinegars will keep indefinitely, although the flavour will lose strength. However, it is generally a good idea to use all vinegar by the date suggested on the label.

If vinegar smells bad or rotten, it should be discarded.

BALSAMIC VINEGAR

Probably one of the most famous of vinegars, 'aceto balsamico' originates from Northern Italy, where it was first fashionable among wealthy 18th-century households.

Balsamic vinegar has been produced in the Italian towns of Modena and Reggio Emilia since the Middle Ages. Barrels of the precious 'balsamico' were originally stored in lofts, where they fermented over some years, then matured for more years, warming up in summer and cooling in winter, gradually evaporating and becoming more concentrated in flavour.

The vinegar is fermented from a must of Trebbiano grapes. Harvested from the Modena or Reggio Emilio areas of Northern Italy, the cooked must is reduced to a dark syrup before it is ready for fermentation using a mother reserved from previous batches. The process of fermentation from the fruit, through alcohol to acetic acid, takes some three years. In the first stage the sugar is converted to alcohol before the vinegar-producing bacteria take over. When the fermentation is complete, then maturation begins. This is no quick process but something that takes many years – from 12 years and upwards, to 50 years or many more for the greatest (and most expensive) vinegars made by this traditional method.

During the process, the vinegar is carefully transferred through a whole series of barrels. The barrels are made from different woods, to impart their character at various stages. It is said that spices may be added at different stages but such ingredients are closely guarded secrets and the barrels and mother of vinegar become treasures that gradually work their magic on successive batches of vinegar. As some vinegar is drawn off the final smaller

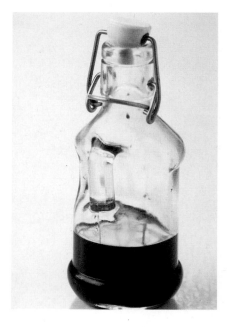

Above: Real 'tradizionale' balsamic vinegar is expensive and should be bought in small quantities and used sparingly.

barrels, so younger stock is moved along and some new vinegar is added to the early barrels to begin its ageing process. This amazing chain of ancient barrels, gradually reducing in size, is preserved and kept working by those who practise traditional balsamic-making methods.

Genuine balsamic vinegar made by this long process is expensive and sold in small quantities. It will be labelled as 'Aceto Balsamico Tradizionale di Modena' or 'Aceto Balsamico Tradizionale di Reggio Emilia', depending on exactly where it was produced.

Balsamic vinegar has been made in this way in Modena and Reggio Emilia since the Middle Ages, and vinegars bearing these labels are protected by the Italian quality assurance label

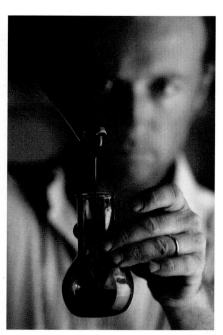

Above: Traditionally produced balsamic vinegars from Modena and Reggio Emilia are aged for at least 12 years.

Above: Methods and ingredients are passed down through generations of vinegar producers and are a strict secret.

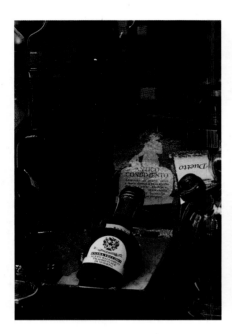

Above: There are many varieties of balsamic vinegar. Check labels for details of ingredients and production methods.

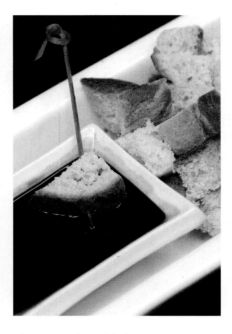

Above: In Italy, rich balsamic vinegar is traditionally served as a dip for fresh white bread before a meal.

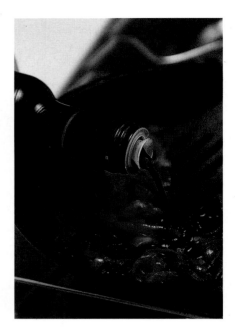

Above: Balsamic vinegar is often used in cooking to deglaze pans after frying or to bring sharpness to a sauce.

'Denominazione di origine controllata' and the European Union's Protected Designation of Origin (PDO). Other balsamic vinegars produced which are not long-aged and do not undergo such strict quality control are simply known as 'aceto balsamico'.

There are all sorts of balsamic vinegars available and the quality varies widely. However, even though less expensive varieties may not be 'proper' balsamic vinegar and nowhere near as fantastic as the traditional, long-aged vinegar, it does not mean they should be dismissed. Think of them as 'balsamic-style' vinegars or vinegar dressings and instead of comparing them in a negative sense with their original source of inspiration, taste them as products in their own right. Some of them are good while others are deeply disappointing. Price is a first guide: a big bottle for very little money is unlikely to be high quality. Check the precise description of the vinegar and the ingredients list to decide whether the bottle contains balsamic vinegar or a sweetened and flavoured vinegar. For example, the product may be a wine vinegar with grape concentrate or a wine vinegar with sugar, fruit juice and caramel.

USE

- As a dip or condiment for bread.
- As a rich dressing, applied by sparing drizzles to individual foods, either savoury or sweet, including fruit.
- For deglazing cooking pans, for example after frying meat or roasting vegetables.
- To enrich sauces and gravies.
- Mixed with water and demerara (raw) sugar as a glaze for meat such as pork or beef.
- To brush over chicken or fish before grilling (broiling)
- In salad dressings.
- To flavour mousses, creams and pâtés.
- To sharpen or enrich drinks, for example with blackcurrant or cranberry juice, topped up with mineral water.
- In some cocktails.
- In smoothies, with fresh fruit, such as strawberries or raspberries.

WHITE BALSAMIC VINEGAR

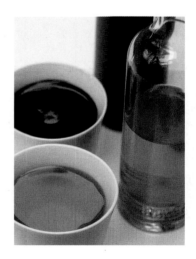

White balsamic vinegars are a good example of products that are not balsamic vinegar at all: check the label and you may find the contents referred to as 'balsamic vinegar condiment'. There are lots of versions on sale of different qualities and prices.

White balsamic vinegar is a mixture of white wine vinegar and white grape must, and does not undergo the same lengthy ageing process as traditional dark balsamic vinegar.

WINE VINEGAR

Red or white wine vinegar, produced by fermenting wine, varies in flavour and quality according to the type of wine, the fermentation process and whether the vinegar has been matured.

Do not automatically assume that all wine vinegars are superior just because they are made from wine – cider vinegar is often a better 'everyday' alternative to inexpensive wine vinegar that can be too harsh and lacking subtle flavours.

Standard, mass-produced inexpensive wine vinegars are unlikely to vary in subtle flavours from one to another, but it is definitely worth sampling different brands, especially among the slightly more expensive ranges, to find one that you prefer.

White and red wine vinegars

All white wine vinegars are light and crisp, and some are very sharp. Red wine vinegars are pink to light red in colour and some are matured, with a stronger, fuller flavour.

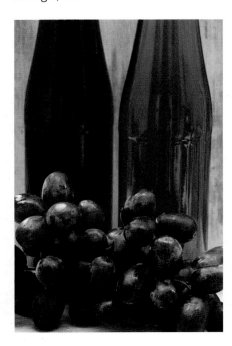

Above: Wine vinegar is the most commonly used vinegar in the Mediterranean.

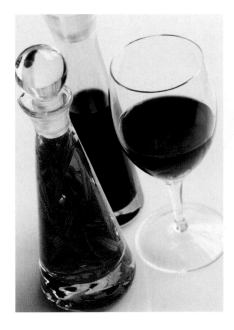

Above: Some wine vinegar is made from a specific wine, such as pinot noir vinegar, or Chardonnay vinegar.

Vinegars made by traditional slow methods and matured have more complex flavours, and their piquancy is rounded or balanced slightly by the fruity tones of the original wine. Sometimes, the depth of flavour comes from the barrel in which the vinegar was aged.

Look for wine vinegars that have been made by the Orléans method, which involves the traditional processes of slow fermentation and maturing. Named wine vinegars will hint at the characteristics of the wine from which they have been fermented. Among the reds, Merlot, Cabernet Sauvignon and pinot noir vinegars are all available. Look out for the wine vinegars of different countries to broaden the tasting experience.

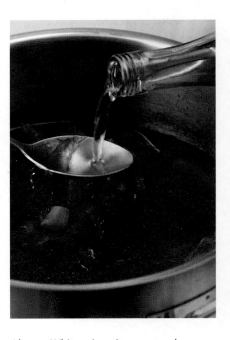

Above: White wine vinegar may be used to sharpen cooking liquor and balance sweet flavours.

USE
- In hot and cold sauces and in salad dressings.
- As a marinade ingredient for white fish or sousing liquid for oily fish.
- In soups, casseroles or stews.
- To sharpen sauce mixtures or drinks.
- For making preserves (it is usually a waste to throw high-quality wine vinegar into a general vegetable pickle or other mixed preserve but less expensive products are suitable).
- For making flavoured vinegars, for example by adding herbs, fruit or spices.
- For home-made natural skin and hair treatments.
- For cleaning and restoring wood (less expensive wine vinegars are most useful for this purpose).

Champagne vinegar

This is made from Champagne and also known as Reims vinegar (vinaigre de Reims), named after the town of Reims, which is centrally located in the Champagne region of France. All Champagne vinegar should be produced here – so check the label.

Champagne vinegar is aged in oak barrels for one year. As a wine vinegar, it is quite sharp but lighter in flavour than white or red wine vinegars. Although, in theory, it should be a superior vinegar, it is worth remembering that its quality depends on the original quality of the wine. A good Champagne vinegar will hint at the pinot noir flavours that are so characteristic of the original wine complemented by the maturing process used for the vinegar.

It is not so long ago that Champagne vinegar was a treat available from specialist shops and wine merchants but it now features among the own-brand products of larger supermarkets.

USE

- For marinades, dressings and sauces, both savoury and sweet.
- In light dressings or to deglaze the cooking pan for fish and shellfish, especially salmon.
- As an accompaniment to oysters.
- To sharpen drinks and desserts, and bring a hint of piquancy to fresh ripe and sweet berries.
- For making delicately flavoured herb, fruit or flower vinegars.
- Drizzled over very sweet ripe peaches.
- To sharpen rich fruit salads or compotes, especially those with dried fruits.
- With nut or truffle oil to make a sublime vinaigrette.

Sherry vinegar

Spain is known for the quality of its sherry vinegars (vinagre de Jerez). Like other wine vinegars, the quality, or blend, of sherries dictates the quality of the vinegar. Good sherry vinegar that is well matured has its sharpness balanced by the full and distinct flavours of the original wine. The best can be mellow

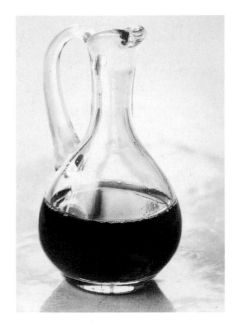

Above: The colour of sherry vinegar varies from golden through to rich dark brown.

and rich, and compared by some to balsamic vinegar. However, as for other vinegars, the flavour depends on the individual product and there are many sherry vinegars available.

USE

- In marinades for red meat, rich poultry and game.
- For bringing a hint of piquancy to rich gravies and sauces, or deglazing cooking pans after frying meat or oily fish.
- For rich salad dressings or cold dressings for meat.
- In soups and pasta sauces.
- In preserves such as pickled shallots.
- Drizzled over grilled (broiled) halloumi cheese or for dressing and marinating cubes of feta or manchego cheese.
- To bring a hint of contrasting piquancy to rich fruit compotes, chocolate syrups, caramel sauces, praline or toffee mixtures.
- For making rich and warming, throat-clearing hot toddies, especially with honey.
- For flavouring rich ice creams, such as brown bread or nut ice creams.

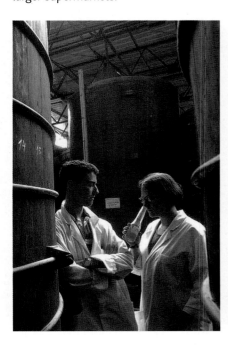

Above: Champagne vinegar is aged in huge oak barrels, and must be produced in the Champagne region of France.

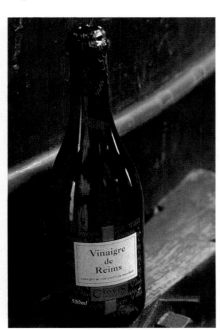

Above: The best quality Champagne vinegars will retain some of the taste of the original Champagne wine.

MALT VINEGAR

Produced in Britain and in other European countries with a history of ale brewing, malt vinegar that is available today is derived from the traditional product 'alegar', or ale vinegar.

Barley, the basic ingredient of malt vinegar, is sprouted, a process that leads to starch being converted to maltose, a type of sugar (not as sweet as sucrose) that develops when starch is digested. Rich, full-flavoured malted barley is fermented to produce alcohol and then onwards to make vinegar. Caramel is added to intensify the flavour and colour of the vinegar. It is important to check the label to ensure that the product is malt vinegar and not an inferior, bitter mixture of diluted acetic acid and caramel or other colouring and flavouring ingredients.

Malt vinegar is famous as the condiment sprinkled on British fish and chips. While some may be horrified at the idea, a little good malt vinegar perfectly complements crisp, hot chips (French fries) and white fish in crunchy batter. Wine vinegar is either too crisp and tart or fruity to cut the flavours to perfection. Malt vinegar is also useful for pickling and making rich chutneys and ketchups. Malt vinegar is sold ready spiced for pickling vegetables, such as onions.

USE
- As a table condiment.
- For making chutneys, pickling and in other savoury preserves.
- As a base for sauces and marinades.
- For household and outdoor use.
- As a general souring agent in cooking, for example in sweet-sour sauces and dishes.

Distilled malt vinegar, white vinegar or spirit vinegar
Distilled malt vinegar is a concentrated malt vinegar with a higher acid content, which makes it ideal for preserving vegetables and other ingredients with a high water content. Water is likely to dilute pickles, making them more vulnerable to attack from micro-organisms. When caramel is not added the distilled vinegar is clear and it may be called white vinegar or distilled white vinegar. The flavour is similar but not as full.

It is important to avoid cheap alternatives that are made by diluting acetic acid with water as they do not have the same flavour as real distilled malt vinegar. Check labels carefully for ingredients – these should consist only of the vinegar and not of acetic acid plus other items. 'Non-brewed condiment' is a term that can be used for this diluted acetic acid.

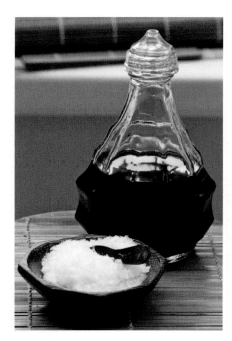

Above: Salt and malt vinegar – the classic accompaniment to British fish and chips.

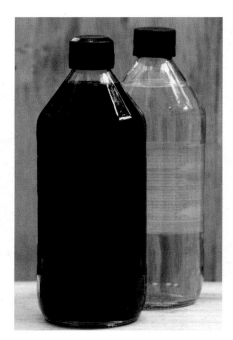

Above: Distilled malt vinegar can be dark brown, or clear if no caramel is added.

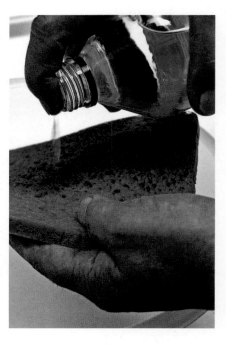

Above: Distilled white vinegar is most economical to use around the home.

USE

- As a pickling vinegar, especially for eggs or light vegetables, such as red cabbage.
- As a raising agent in baking.
- For first aid – such as treating bites or stings.
- For household and outdoor use.

Light malt vinegar

This is a pale gold-coloured vinegar brewed as for ordinary malt vinegar but without the addition of caramel. The flavour is milder and very similar in taste to rice vinegar.

USE

- As a pickling vinegar when a milder flavour is required.
- For salad dressings and sauces.
- In marinades for meat, poultry or fish.
- To sharpen drinks.
- As a raising agent in baking.

Pickling vinegar

This is distilled malt vinegar flavoured with a mix of spices typically used for pickling vegetables. It may be dark malt vinegar or white vinegar, but in

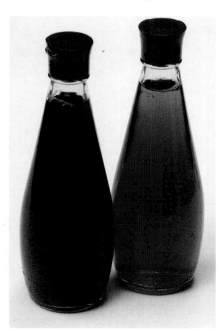

Above: Light malt vinegar has a milder taste than ordinary malt vinegar.

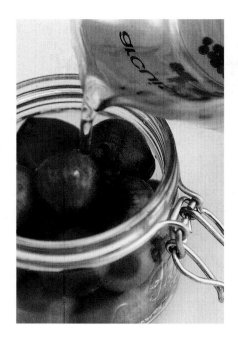

Above: Onions are often pickled in malt vinegar which has been spiced with peppercorns, cloves and chillies.

both cases the flavour of the spices is usually very mild. Black peppercorns, coriander seeds, ginger, allspice, cloves, mustard seeds, dried red chillies and cinnamon may all be used to spice vinegar for pickling. To impart a more distinct flavour when pickling, it is best to infuse the whole spices in plain malt vinegar. When spicing your own vinegar at home, malt, wine and cider vinegars can all be used.

USE

- In light fruit chutneys (such as peach, pear or apricot) or for making fruit or herb jellies, such as apple or mint jelly.
- For pickling onions, red cabbage, chillis, cucumbers, beetroot (beet) or hard-boiled eggs.
- To make sweet fruit pickles (sugar should be dissolved in the vinegar to sweeten it slightly).
- In sweet-sour braised vegetables, such as red cabbage, when vinegar is lightly spiced.
- In punchy salad dressings, for example to dress meat salads.

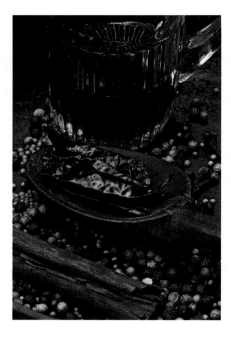

Above: Ready-spiced pickling vinegar is available to buy, but it is very easy to make using malt, wine or cider vinegar.

MAKING SPICED VINEGAR

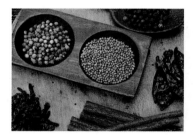

Place 1 cinnamon stick, 12 cloves, 60ml/4 tbsp coriander seeds, 30 ml/2 tbsp mustard seeds and 15 ml/1 tbsp black peppercorns in a large heavy pan.

Place over a medium heat, shaking the pan often, until the spices are lightly roasted and giving off their aroma. Do not overcook the spices until they begin to pop or brown. Add 4 dried red chillies and pour in a little vinegar taken from 2.4 litres/4 pints/10 cups malt vinegar, adding enough to cover the spices generously.

Bring to the boil, then remove from the heat and pour in the remaining vinegar. Cover tightly and leave to infuse for 1–5 days. Strain the vinegar into clean bottles and cover tightly, then store in a cool place.

CIDER VINEGAR

One of the oldest and original cottage-industry vinegars, apple cider vinegar is still renowned for its health benefits; it is also one of the most useful of culinary vinegars.

One of the traditional vinegars made in apple-growing areas, and well known especially in the US and Great Britain, cider vinegar is an ancient cure-all that has retained its reputation as a healing agent and general health-giving potion. Cider vinegar is said to make a positive contribution to everything from weight-loss and relieving arthritis to reducing cholesterol levels and the prevention of heart disease. It is available to purchase in pharmacies and healthfood shops, as well as in supermarkets. Many people swear by a daily dose of cider vinegar for general wellbeing, while others employ it as a beauty product. It is also one of the most versatile of culinary vinegars.

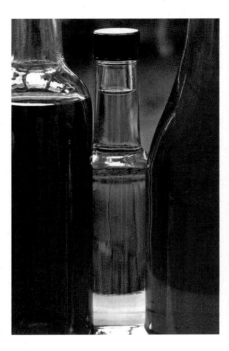

Above: Cider vinegar varies in colour, from colourless or very pale yellow to a rich gold, and can be cloudy or clear.

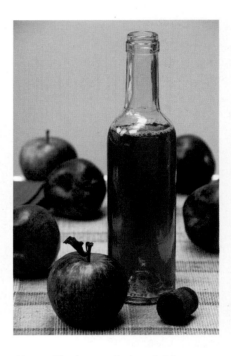

Above: The best varieties of cider vinegar are made from just one type of apple.

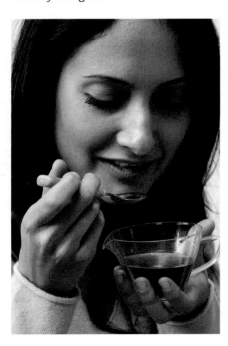

Above: Cider vinegar is prized for its health benefits. Drinking a teaspoon a day is said to help all manner of ailments.

Cider vinegar is made from apples, starting with the raw fruit, fruit juice, apple wine or cider. There are delicate, yet distinct apple-like flavours in some cider vinegars. The best, and most expensive, vinegars are made from single types of apples. Unsurprisingly, the quality of the base product influences the quality of vinegar and there is a very large selection from which to choose. Cloudy vinegars that contain some fruit residue may not look as appealing, but they are often superior in taste. There are both organic and unpasteurized cider vinegars, made by fast or slow methods, from small or large producers. The choice can be overwhelming. Read the labels on cider vinegar bottles to check if there are any added ingredients or if the product is an inferior blend of vinegar or acetic acid with apple juice.

As a general rule, cider vinegar is milder than other wine and malt vinegars; some are clear, others cloudy, and the colour of the different types varies from pale yellow to a honey-like gold.

CIDER VINEGAR STARTER

Many varieties of live organic cider vinegar are available. These can be used as a starting point for experiments with making vinegar at home. It should be added to live organic cider or wine.

Live organic cider vinegar

When using cider vinegar for its health benefits, it is important to select an organic product, which is made from the fruit (rather than vinegar plus juice), preferably live, without any added chemicals to 'kill off' the vinegar bacteria.

Cider vinegar must be stored in an airtight container in a cool, dark place to preserve any vitamin C it may contain. Buy modest quantities rather than large amounts so that it will be used within the date indicated on the bottle.

As well as for internal health benefits, the fruit acids and residues in this vinegar are helpful in home-made beauty products, for example as an exfoliator to remove dead skin residue and as a face freshener.

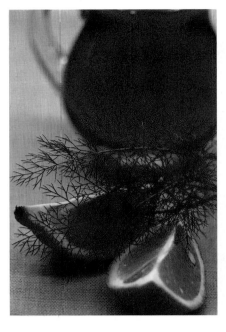

Above: On its own, or with other ingredients, cider vinegar can be used to make natural home remedies.

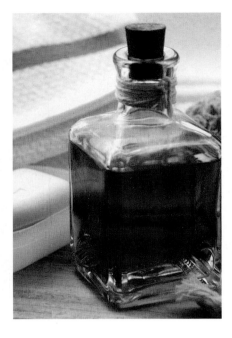

Above: Using cider vinegar on the skin after bathing can help to redress any imbalance in the skin's pH levels.

Diet and cider vinegar

Cider vinegar has been associated with weight-loss, with claims that drinking it helps to reduce fat absorption or even break down fat in the body. Cider vinegar tablets or capsules are sold in healthfood stores as a natural slimming aid. While there is no scientific evidence to support the digestive theories, including cider vinegar as part of a balanced diet is a good idea, especially if it encourages a taste for less-sweet, less-rich foods and when it is used in beverages that replace high-sugar drinks.

USE

- As a home remedy or preventative agent for promoting good health.
- For first-aid, such as treating insect bites or stings.
- To soothe tired muscles and aches and pains by adding a little to a warm bath.
- For home-made beauty treatments such as hair rinses and face packs.
- As a base for home-made vinegar.
- As a cleaning agent around the home.
- In salad dressings, sauces and dips.
- In relishes and salsas.
- To bring piquancy to a wide variety of savoury or sweet dishes without making them too harsh.
- In sweet dishes such as sorbets, ice creams and mousses.
- For drinks and cordials.
- In smoothies – try a quick cider vinegar and banana smoothie by whizzing up a banana and yogurt in a blender then drizzling in a little cider vinegar for a zesty flavour.
- In some preserves and pickles.
- As a base for home-made flavoured vinegars, particularly herb vinegars.

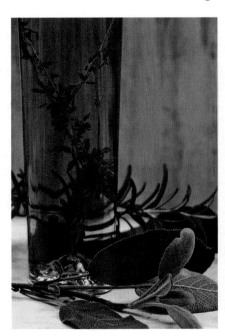

Above: The mild taste of cider vinegar makes it a very good base for home-made herb-flavoured vinegars.

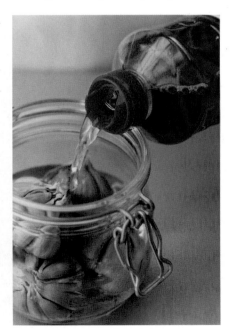

Above: Cider vinegar is often used to pickle ingredients with a strong flavour, such as garlic or shallots.

RICE VINEGAR

An essential part of Asian cuisine for centuries, many types of rice vinegar and rice vinegar dressings are now available in specialist and healthfood stores as well as supermarkets.

Rice vinegars may be fermented either from rice or from rice wine. Traditional methods started with the process of fermenting the rice itself, rather than making rice wine into vinegar. Rice vinegars vary in colour and flavour; some are milder than wine vinegar or malt vinegar while others are harsher and more comparable with light malt vinegar. Some of the rice vinegars available are sweetened or flavoured and coloured, so it is worth checking the ingredients on the label carefully.

As well as the familiar Asian rice vinegars, Californian rice vinegars are also available. They are made from grain harvested locally and include organic brown rice vinegars, which can be plain or seasoned. Brown rice vinegar can have a very strong and distinctive flavour, which is more noticeable than that of the majority of wine or malt vinegars.

Chinese rice vinegars range in colour from clear to various shades of red and brown, through to black. In Chinese medicine, rice vinegar is used in soup that is recommended to ease asthma. It is also thought to be clearing, helpful for good digestion and useful for promoting liver and stomach function. It is also believed to help external conditions of the skin.

As a rule, Japanese rice vinegar, or su, is lighter than Chinese vinegar. It is available in many varieties and qualities. Traditionally brewed vinegars made from unpolished glutinous rice have a reputation for good quality. Notice the difference between rice vinegar and rice vinegar dressing, as

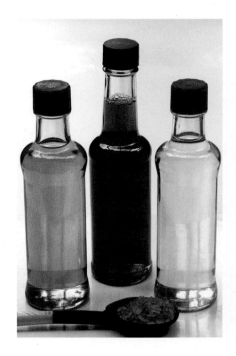

Above: Rice vinegars vary in colour, from clear, through to amber-yellow and red.

the latter will be seasoned and sweetened or flavoured, for example, ready for mixing with sushi rice. Vinegared rice, or su-meshi, is made by dressing cooked rice with a mixture of rice vinegar, sugar and salt.

Rice vinegar may be flavoured with Japanese citrus fruit, such as dai dai, a type of bitter orange. Ready-made, this sauce is sold as ponzu in Japan.

Black rice vinegar

Popular in southern China, black rice vinegar has a full flavour and may be enriched with malt. Black vinegar may be aged and intense in flavour. Chinkiang vinegar, which originated in the city of Zhenjiang in the eastern coastal province of

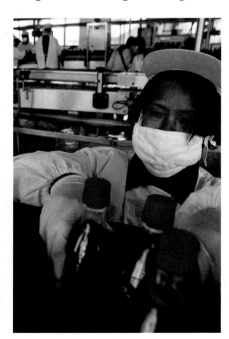

Above: Black rice vinegar is popular in Japan, where it is sold in health drinks.

Above: Bottles of Chinkiang vinegar are checked on the production line.

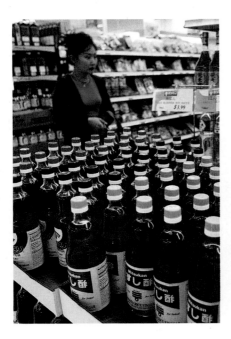

Above: A wide variety of rice vinegars can be found in Asian supermarkets. They vary in taste and quality.

Jiangsu in China, has a reputation as being one of the best. The longer the vinegar is kept, the stronger its aroma becomes. As with other superior varieties of vinegars, there are always inexpensive alternatives of inferior quality, so it is worth experimenting to find a good product.

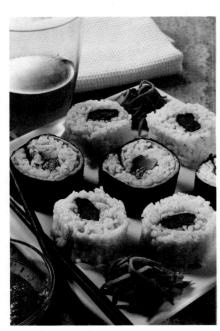

Above: Japanese rice vinegar is an essential part of sushi preparation.

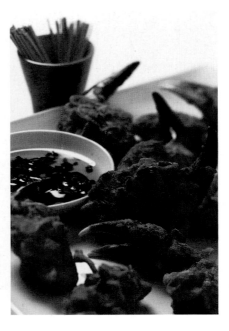

Above: Black, red and white rice vinegars are often used in dipping sauces in Asian cuisine.

In Japan, black rice vinegar (kurozu) is prized for its health benefits, and in recent years has been sold in vinegar drinks which are available from supermarkets and vending machines, as well as from dedicated vinegar bars.

USE

- In meat dishes as a marinade and tenderizing agent.
- As a dipping sauce.
- As a substitute for balsamic vinegar.
- In soups and sauces.
- In stir-fries.
- In health drinks.

Red rice vinegar

This varies from a lighter variety of black rice vinegar to a seasoned, sweet and full-flavoured vinegar that is popular as a dipping sauce or for adding to soups.

USE

- As a substitute for black vinegar – just add a little sugar.
- As a dipping sauce.
- In noodles, soup and seafood dishes.

White rice vinegar

This is colourless or a very pale yellow colour, light in flavour, with different regional variations or specialities.

USE

- To dress vegetables and salads.
- In sweet-and-sour dishes or hot-and-sour recipes, such as the classic soup.
- For making refreshing drinks.
- For dressing rice and in Japanese sushi.
- As a pickling medium, for example, for garlic or ginger.
- In Western cooking, in salad dressings, sauces and drinks.
- In both hot and cold sauces, including dipping sauces and sweet-and-sour sauces.

MAKING SUSHI RICE

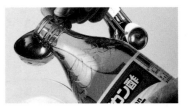

Vinegared rice (su-meshi) is the essential base for all kinds of sushi. Put 200g/7oz/ 1 cup Japanese short grain rice in a large bowl and wash in plenty of water, until it runs clear. Tip into a sieve (strainer) and leave to drain for 1 hour.

Put the rice into a small, deep pan with 15 per cent more water, i.e. 250ml/8fl oz/1⅕ cups water to 200g/7oz/1 cup rice. Cover and bring to the boil. This takes about 5 minutes. Reduce the heat and simmer for 12 minutes without lifting the lid. You should hear a faint crackling noise. The rice should now have absorbed the water. Remove from the heat and leave for 10 minutes.

Transfer the cooked rice to a wet Japanese rice tub or bowl. Mix 40ml/ 8 tsp rice vinegar with 20ml/4 tsp caster (superfine) sugar and 5ml/1 tsp salt, until dissolved. Add to the rice, fluffing with a wet spatula. Cover the bowl with a wet dish towel and leave to cool.

OTHER VINEGARS

Vinegar can be made from many ingredients. Fermented fruit vinegars are popular around the world, while coconut, cane and palm vinegars are used predominantly in South-east Asia.

Vinegar is a global ingredient, used in the cooking of almost every cuisine, as well as for health, beauty and household purposes. It has traditionally been made from whatever ingredients are grown locally.

Fermented fruit vinegar

As well as wine and cider vinegars originating from grapes and apples, many other varieties of fruit are involved in the vinegar fermentation process. Vinegars made from fermented fruit are different from fruit-flavoured vinegars, where fruit are macerated in a vinegar to impart their flavour to it. Fermented fruit vinegars are expensive, and usually produced in relatively modest quantities. A wide variety of fruit may be used, including familiar raspberries, but also tomatoes, blueberries, pears, quinces, pineapple, bananas, peaches or apricots. Plums, fresh or dried, are also used. Many of these vinegars will retain the flavour of the original fruit. Most fresh fruit vinegars are produced in Europe, but persimmon vinegar is often used in Korean cooking (as well as apple-based cider vinegars).

As well as fresh fruit, dried fruit, such as raisins, currants, dates or figs, can be used to make richly flavoured vinegars. Raisin vinegar is used in Middle Eastern cooking and is a cloudy brown colour, with a mild taste. Dried fruit vinegars are predominantly produced in countries such as Turkey, Greece, Spain, Morocco and Algeria.

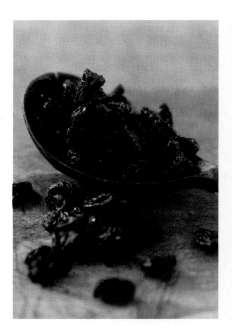

Above: Vinegar fermented from raisins is popular in the Middle Eastern countries, where it is used in cooking.

The best fermented fruit vinegars are aromatic, carrying the distinct flavour of the fruit in a well-balanced vinegar that is acidic and fruity but not sweetened. These products are expensive and a vinegar treat rather than a store-cupboard staple.

USE
- As dressings for individual ingredients – light fruit vinegars are best for this.
- In marinades for meat, poultry or fish.
- To dress fresh fruit.
- In desserts and drinks.
- Drizzled over light cheeses, such as mozzarella or soft goat's cheese.
- To enrich savoury sauces or casseroles. Rich fruit vinegars may be paired with meat dishes.
- With nut oils for rich salad dressings.

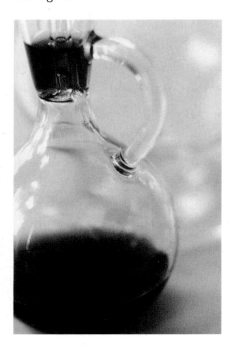

Above: Fig vinegar, as well as vinegar fermented from raisins and dates, is used in Mediterranean countries.

Above: Raspberry vinegar has a distinctive red colour and can be quite sweet if sugar has been added.

Coconut vinegar

This is made from fermented coconut water (the clear liquid naturally occurring in coconuts, not to be confused with coconut milk, which is made from the flesh of the fruit). Coconut vinegar is very popular in South-east Asian cuisine, particularly in the Philippines. It is a cloudy white vinegar, with a slight flavour of yeast.

In Filipino cooking, ingredients are often marinated in coconut vinegar, ginger and garlic before cooking, and raw ingredients such as oily fish and shrimp are cured in lime juice and coconut vinegar, as is exemplified in the national favourite kinilaw (Filipino cured herring).

The Filipino penchant for sweet and sour notes is achieved by combining coconut vinegar or kalamansi lime juice with palm sugar (jaggery) or cane sugar, as in adobo (chicken and pork cooked with vinegar and ginger), the national dish, which originally hailed from Mexico.

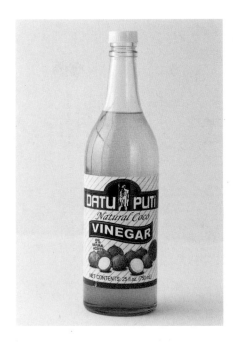

Above: In the Philippines, coconut vinegar is used extensively. It can be found in speciality stores.

USE

- In South-east Asian dishes, such as stews, for authentic flavour.
- As a marinade for meat, poultry and fish dishes.
- In sauces and soups.
- To cure fish and shellfish.

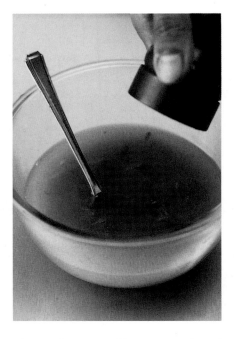

Above: Filipino cured herring is marinated in coconut vinegar mixed with lime juice, and flavoured with ginger and chillies.

Cane vinegar

Made from fermented sugar cane, this is popular in the Philippines. The colour varies from pale yellow to dark brown, and it has a mild flavour, not unlike rice vinegar. There is no trace of sweetness in the vinegar from the sugar cane.

USE

- In salads and sauces, or as a glaze for cooked meats.
- In vinaigrettes when combined with rich nut oils such as walnut oil.

Palm vinegar

This cloudy white vinegar is made from the fermented sap from the fruit of the nipa palm. It looks similar to coconut vinegar, but has a milder taste. Also popular in the Philippines, it is milder than wine or cider vinegars.

USE

- In dipping sauces with chilli and garlic.
- As a dressing for salads and vegetables.
- As a marinade for meat, poultry or fish.
- In soups and sauces.

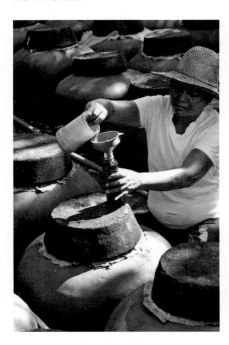

Above: A sugar cane farmer in the Philippines tests the sugar cane juice which is fermenting in earthenware jars.

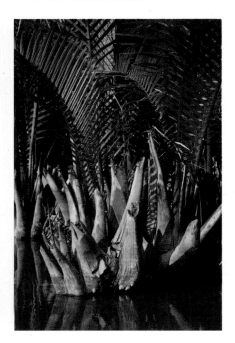

Above: The fruit of the nipa palm produces a sap which is fermented to make alcohol and palm vinegar.

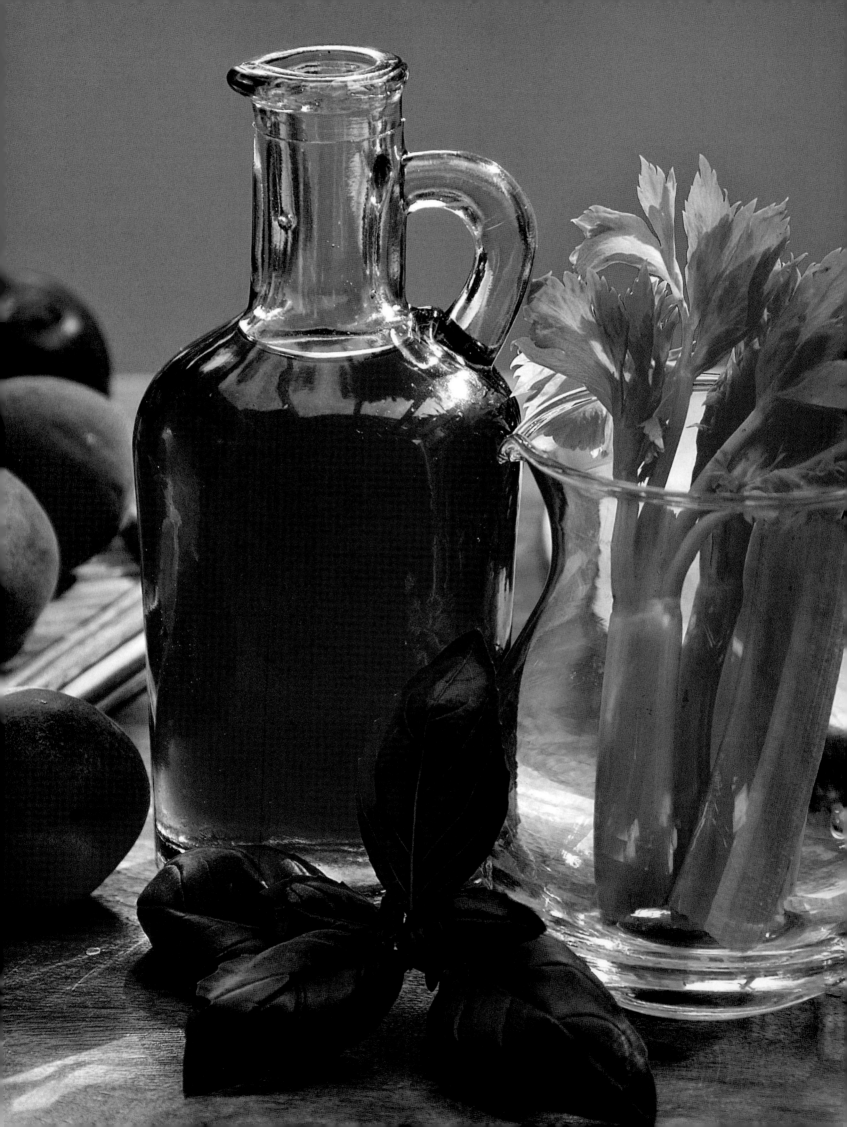

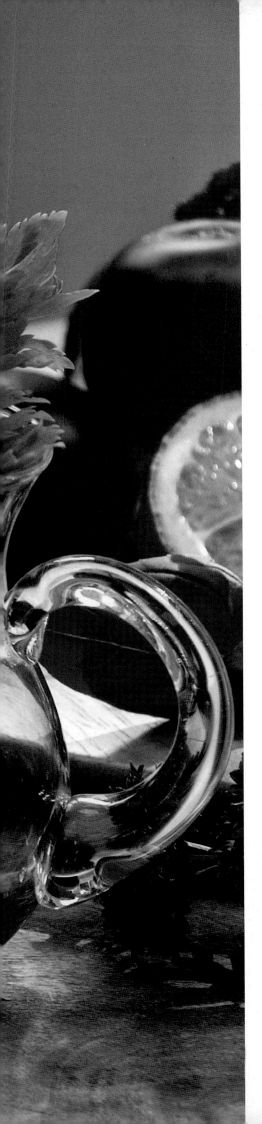

VINEGAR FOR HEALTH AND HEALING

This section provides a selection of ideas that make the most of vinegar's health-giving properties. Cider vinegar is particularly appreciated in a wide variety of uses for promoting positive health and healing: from an antiseptic agent or external coolant to an internal provider of holistic help for long-term wellbeing. A little vinegar may be taken regularly as a refreshing ingredient in health-promoting drinks. It is also a great standby for first aid use when a simple home cure is sufficient.

Left: Alongside a healthy diet and regular exercise, vinegar contributes to general good health and wellbeing and is used to treat specific ailments.

VINEGAR AS A TONIC

Before modern antiseptics, drugs, vitamin pills and medicines became everyday potions, vinegar, especially cider vinegar, was widely used to promote good health.

Vinegar has been used for its health benefits for centuries. The positive effect that vinegar is said to have on a range of chronic diseases continues to be supported. Many people assert that their symptoms are reduced by taking regular doses of vinegar. Cider vinegar in particular has been taken for many years as a general health tonic as well as to treat specific ailments. However, modern medical theories cannot offer a precise explanation for why and how vinegar works. The general nutritional benefits and its influence on eating patterns are likely factors, but there is greater evidence for the dietary role that vinegar can play in supporting the acid-alkali balance in the body.

WHICH VINEGAR TO USE?

Organic cider vinegar is generally recommended for remedies and as a tonic. There are also different flavoured organic vinegars based on cider vinegar, including raspberry vinegar, that are excellent for drinks and dressings. It is also worth looking out for natural, live vinegars fermented from fruit, such as raspberry and blueberry vinegars, as they provide the goodness from the particular type of fruit, just as cider vinegar does from apples.

Cider vinegar is also the recommended choice for external treatments, for example it can be used for treating mild skin conditions as well as for making pleasant rinses and washes, but other types, such as malt or rice vinegar, are also useful for their health benefits.

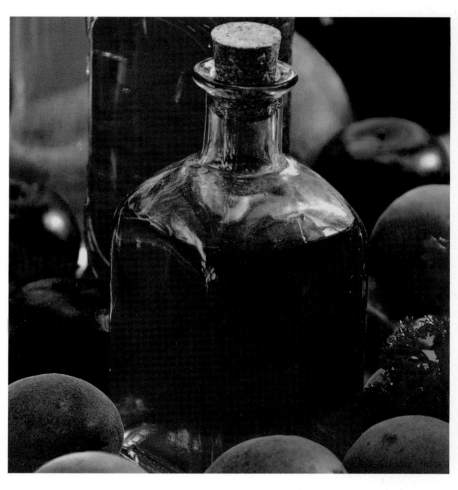

Above: Vinegar can make a positive contribution to health when part of a balanced diet.

Ancient harmony and health

Vinegar was prescribed in ancient times to support natural harmony or balance. The ancient Greek physician Hippocrates recommended vinegar for clearing and cleansing the system and functions associated with the kidneys and liver. Vinegar is one of many ingredients still used in Chinese medicine for promoting good health through diet. It is also believed to help arrest bleeding, aid digestion, combat parasites, treat jaundice, skin complaints and nose bleeds.

Vinegar and nutrients

The nutritional value of vinegar depends on the ingredients from which it is made. Typically, vinegar contains minerals, especially potassium, as well as some chloride, phosphorus, magnesium, sodium and sulphur, with a little calcium and traces of other minerals. Minerals are important in modest amounts and are widely distributed among foods. Although the proportions are not high in vinegar compared to the main ingredients used in meals, vinegar

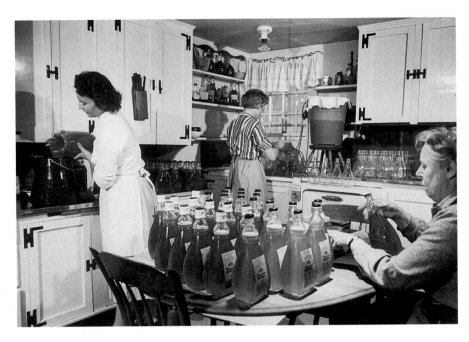

Above: In 1950s America, a mixture of vinegar and honey called 'Honegar' was marketed as a cure-all elixir. There are still many people who swear by the healing powers of vinegar.

makes a helpful contribution when it is used regularly. Vinegar is a valuable flavouring and seasoning ingredient, in cooked dishes, dressings, sauces and drinks.

The acid-alkali balance

For healthy, normal function the body has to maintain an important acid-alkali balance. Gastric juices are acidic so that they can digest food, but the acids must not enter the digestive system. The body has an efficient buffer system that keeps the cells at the required levels. Deficiencies and health problems are often reflected by changes in the pH levels in the body and these have to be rectified, both in the short term and by long-term control. Eating the right diet helps to rectify poor balance because some foods are acid-forming while others are neutral or alkaline-forming. Vinegar is a neutral to slightly alkaline-forming food.

Whether a food is acid- or alkaline-forming depends on its nutritional make-up and what effect it has during digestion. For example, acid-forming foods include fish, meat and eggs, dairy products, refined starches and sugary foods. Fruit and vegetables are generally alkaline-forming. Eating 80 per cent alkaline-forming and 20 per cent acid-forming foods is recommended as a general rule. Eating foods that create an acidic environment encourages the body to secrete alkaline substances into the blood, maintaining the balance.

The power of cider vinegar

This has long been regarded as a 'cure-all'. Natural, unpasteurized, cider vinegar made by traditional methods is thought to be beneficial for the pectin it contains from the apples. Pectin, a form of soluble fibre also found in other ingredients, such as oats, can help to maintain healthy blood cholesterol levels.

Consumed regularly, there is much evidence that vinegar (in particular cider vinegar) helps to relieve joint pain associated with arthritis. Vinegar also helps to promote a healthy cardiovascular system, including good blood cholesterol levels and blood pressure.

Vinegar is useful for protecting against general colds and helping to relieve cold symptoms. It promotes good digestion, helps to reduce and avoid indigestion and to relieve diarrhoea. As a short-term tonic it can help to cleanse the system as part of a process of detoxing intended to promote good liver function.

It is also useful as a general tonic for promoting a sense of wellbeing. Warm cider vinegar drinks can help to promote sleep.

Anyone suffering from a medical condition should take professional medical advice before introducing new foods into the diet or making any diet changes which are intended to alleviate symptoms. Aside from using vinegar as a home remedy for minor conditions, for anyone who is active and healthy, using cider vinegar as a tonic or everyday ingredient in drinks or daily cooking is a great way of promoting good health. To be effective, regular use of cider vinegar should be part of a general diet and lifestyle review that should be planned and seen as a long term change.

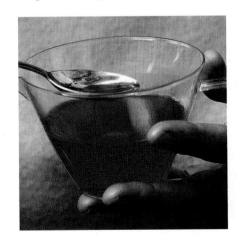

Above: Vinegar can be taken internally to help a variety of complaints.

VINEGAR FOR HEALING

A small bottle of vinegar makes a handy addition to any first aid kit or bathroom cabinet. It can be used on its own or with other ingredients to treat many common ailments.

The natural acidic and astringent properties of vinegar mean that it can be effective as a disinfectant, antiseptic and coolant. It is a good idea to keep a small bottle of vinegar in the bathroom, where it will be useful for treating a variety of complaints. It is very good for cleansing cuts and scrapes in the first instance.

External use of vinegar

Cider vinegar contains alpha-hydroxy acids, or natural fruit acids, which are very good for the skin. It makes a fantastic natural exfoliator, on its own or mixed with other ingredients. It can be used in washes and rinses or applied directly to skin, either neat or diluted, to calm and cleanse skin conditions and infections, including acne and blocked pores.

Cider vinegar is a good choice for treating skin problems, but other types of vinegar, in particular malt and rice vinegar, are also effective. They are useful neat or diluted as astringents, as well as an antiseptics for clearing simple outbreaks of spots. A little neat vinegar on a cotton wool ball can be applied to spots to clean the area and prevent further infection.

Vinegar is a simple and effective antiseptic for cleaning up minor cuts and grazes, and can be used for cooling and cleansing insect bites, wasp stings and jellyfish stings. In parts of northern Australia where box jellyfish are common, vinegar is even provided on beaches so it can be applied quickly to stings while

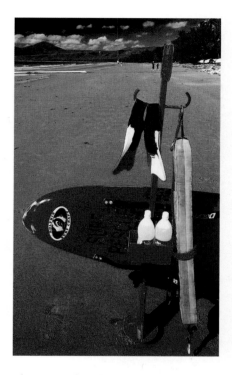

Above: Bottles of vinegar form part of an Australian lifeguard's equipment – vinegar is used to treat jellyfish stings.

waiting for medical treatment. The acetic acid in vinegar is said to disable any venom that has not yet entered the bloodstream. Box jellyfish stings can be fatal to humans, so proper medical attention must be sought.

As well as treating their bites and stings, vinegar can also be used as a repellent to keep insects, including mosquitoes, away. Transferring a small amount of vinegar to a spray bottle is a great way of creating a natural insect spray that will not be harmful to children or pets.

Vinegar is helpful for clearing infestations of head lice and for resolving mild dandruff problems. For healthy feet, vinegar can be used

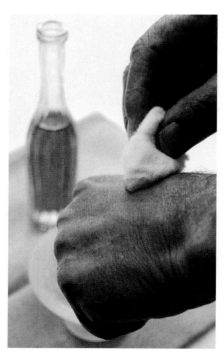

Above: Cider vinegar can be applied directly to the skin to treat skin conditions.

Above: Vinegar is a natural antiseptic. Use to soothe and calm minor irritations.

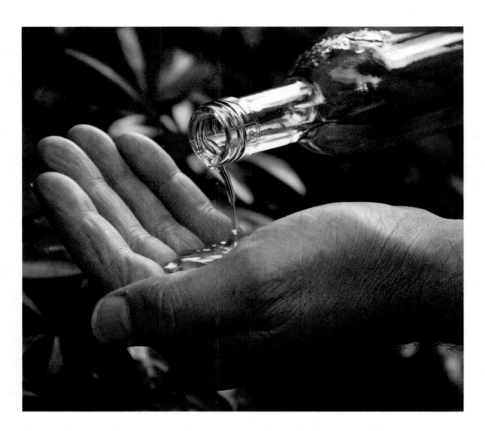

Above: The natural properties of vinegar mean that it has been used for many centuries as a disinfectant, antiseptic and general health tonic.

in the removal of corns or for overcoming common fungal infections, such as athlete's foot. It is also good for reducing soreness and swelling and for soothing dry or itchy skin.

Vinegar baths or soaks can help to relieve tired and aching muscles, and to reduce the soreness of bruising, as well as to cool sunburn. Minor burns can be treated by dabbing on a little neat vinegar.

Vinegar steam baths are useful for clearing a blocked-up nose and other symptoms of a head cold. Mixed with honey, another natural antiseptic, and different herbs, vinegar makes a very effective gargle to soothe a sore throat.

Vinegar in natural remedies

Use simple homely treatments for minor ailments that do not pose any significant threat to health.

For example, many of the vinegar remedies suggested here are perfect to soothe the symptoms of common illnesses such as coughs and colds.

Wellbeing is defined as part of good health. Some of the vinegar remedies and drinks in this book are very useful for anyone who is run down or stressed. Such simple remedies are often sufficient to prevent a condition from developing. It is important to recognize progress and relief of symptoms or acknowledge the need for medical help.

Make any changes gradually and they are more likely to be enduring and effective. With a diagnosed condition or illness, you should never dismiss medical advice and entirely reject prescribed drugs. It is important to differentiate between vital treatment and complementary, holistic and dietary changes with the help of a doctor.

MAKING FOUR THIEVES VINEGAR

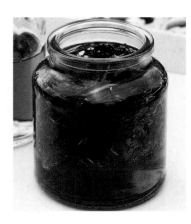

During an outbreak of plague in medieval France, a gang of four thieves, who made a living by robbing the bodies of the dead, were said to avoid succumbing to the disease themselves by making liberal use of a strong herbal vinegar. Many versions of the recipe have been attributed to them. This formula, based on an amalgam of the old recipes, is effective as a mild antiseptic, or to take in prophylactic doses of 5ml/1 tsp, two or three times daily, when exposed to colds and other infections.

Ingredients
15ml/1 tbsp each dried lavender, rosemary, sage and peppermint
2–3 bay leaves
10ml/2 tsp dried wormwood
5ml/1 tsp garlic granules
5ml/1 tsp ground cloves
5ml/1 tsp ground cinnamon
600ml/1 pint/2½ cups cider vinegar

1 Put all the dry ingredients into a jar together and mix. Fill the jar with cider vinegar.

2 Cover tightly and leave in a warm place, such as a sunny windowsill or by a boiler, for 10 days.

3 Strain off the vinegar, through a sieve (strainer) lined with kitchen paper, into a clean jug, then pour it into a sterilized bottle and seal.

Caution
Do not take internally for longer than 2 weeks at a time. Do not take if pregnant, as wormwood is a uterine stimulant.

VINEGAR DRINKS FOR HEALTH

These vinegar drinks are refreshing, reinvigorating and restoring. Simply add a spoonful of vinegar to a glass of water, or mix with other ingredients.

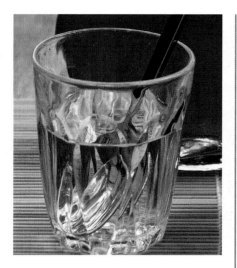

Indigestion

Cider vinegar contains pectin, which is good for digestion. It also acts as an antiseptic in the intestines.

Add 5ml/1 tsp cider vinegar to a small glass of water (about 175ml/6fl oz/ ¾ cup) and mix well. Drink this daily to relieve indigestion.

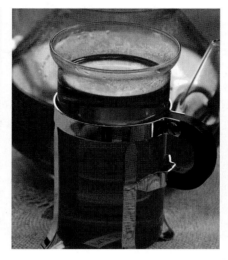

Asthma

In Chinese medicine, vinegar is one of the ingredients believed to help treat asthma. Vinegar is used in drinks and in soup (for example hot-and-sour soup).

Add 5ml/1 tsp vinegar to 250ml/8fl oz/ 1 cup of hot water. Drink daily to help with the symptoms of asthma.

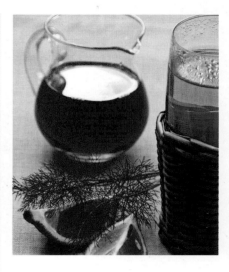

Stress

Fennel, vinegar and lemon tea makes a good mid-morning stress buster or afternoon pick-me-up. Fennel tea is available from health stores.

Add 5ml/1 tsp cider vinegar and a squeeze of fresh lemon juice to a cup of hot fennel tea.

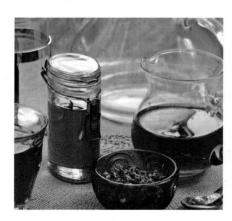

Tension

Camomile tea, apple juice, cider vinegar and honey makes a soothing drink.

Add 5ml/1 tsp each of cider vinegar and honey and 15ml/1 tbsp apple juice to a cup of calming camomile tea.

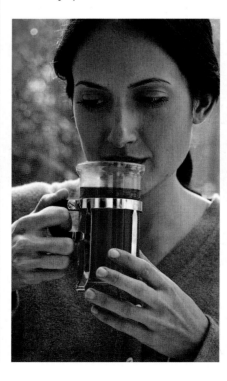

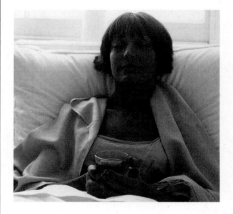

Insomnia

A cider vinegar and honey drink before bed helps to promote calm and can help combat insomnia.

Mix 10ml/2 tsp cider vinegar with 10ml/ 2 tsp honey and top up with warm water.

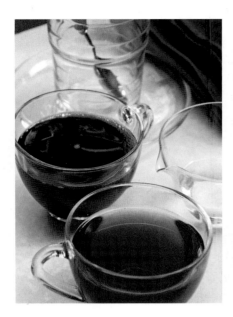

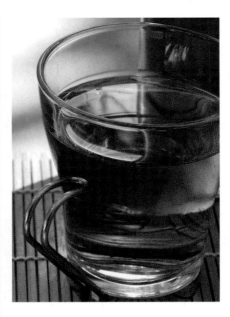

A SPOONFUL OF VINEGAR

Just one spoonful of vinegar can make a difference to your health. It can be taken neat, or diluted in a glass of water.

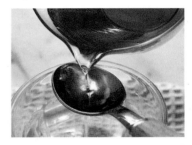

WAXY EAR BUILD-UP Mix 15ml/1 tbsp each of white distilled vinegar and warm water and use as a gentle ear wash to remove any waxy build-up. Do not use this technique if you are suffering (or have suffered) from an ear infection or inflammation.

DIARRHOEA This is the body's natural way of eliminating toxins from the body. It can also be a symptom of a wide range of complaints. If your symptoms persist, seek professional advice. Cider vinegar will alleviate the intensity of diarrhoea but will not stop it completely. Take 5ml/1 tsp cider vinegar in a glass of water, approximately six times a day, before meals and in between.

IRRITABLE BOWEL SYNDROME Add 5ml/1 tsp of cider vinegar to a glass of water. Drink daily to relieve the symptoms.

CONSTIPATION Cider vinegar contains pectin, which can help your body maintain regular bowel movements. Take 5ml/1 tsp daily.

HICCUPS Try drinking a 5ml/1 tsp of cider vinegar to cure hiccups. If the attack of hiccups is particularly severe, try gargling with cider vinegar.

HEARTBURN This usually occurs 1–2 hours after eating. Drinking 5ml/1 tsp cider vinegar in a glass of water before a meal can help to prevent.

HEART HEALTH The potassium in cider vinegar helps to maintain a healthy heart and blood pressure.

Cholesterol

The grape juice and vinegar in this drink contain properties which may help to lower cholesterol levels.

INGREDIENTS

250ml/8fl oz/1 cup red grape juice

120ml/4fl oz/½ cup apple juice

20ml/4 tsp white distilled vinegar

1 Pour the red grape juice and apple juice into a large glass.

2 Add the white distilled vinegar to the glass, stir and chill for at least 1 hour in the refrigerator.

3 Drink a little of the mixture before main meals to help reduce cholesterol levels.

Lethargy

Cider vinegar, honey, mint and orange make an uplifting drink for anyone suffering from fatigue.

INGREDIENTS

475ml/16fl oz/2 cups water

6–8 fresh mint leaves

30ml/2 tbsp fresh orange juice

5ml/1 tsp cider vinegar

5ml/1 tsp honey

1 Bring the water to the boil in a small pan and add the fresh mint leaves.

2 Simmer for 2 minutes, remove from the heat, strain, and add the orange juice, cider vinegar and honey.

3 Serve warm or cool and serve chilled.

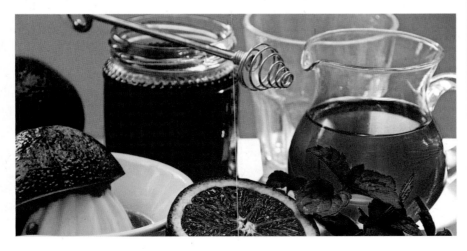

VINEGAR REMEDIES FOR COUGHS AND COLDS

Cider vinegar and honey are classic partners in the fight against everyday minor infections – soothing sore throats and blocked sinuses and assisting recovery.

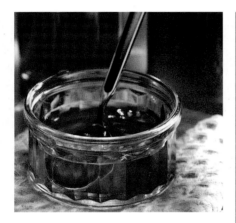

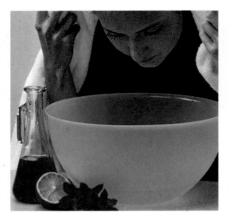

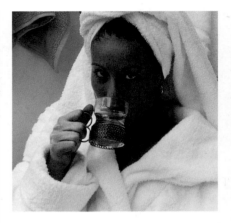

Coughs and sore throat

Cider vinegar and honey both have natural antiseptic qualities so are excellent for relieving and soothing coughs and sore throats.

INGREDIENTS
30ml/2 tbsp cider vinegar
30ml/2 tbsp honey

1 Place the cider vinegar and honey in a small bowl and mix together well.

2 Take the occasional teaspoonful as needed to ease the irritation of a cough or sore throat.

Health tip
Try stirring the honey and vinegar mixture into a cup of hot water for a soothing drink.

VINEGAR GARGLE
Adding 15ml/1 tbsp cider vinegar to a cup of lukewarm water makes a good antiseptic gargle to help relieve a sore throat. Use this to complement cider vinegar and honey soothing drinks.

Blocked sinuses

A combination of cider vinegar, lemon juice and fresh mint leaves is both warming and clearing when a cold or blocked sinuses make breathing difficult.

INGREDIENTS
boiling water
juice of ½ lemon
small bunch fresh mint leaves
30ml/2 tbsp cider vinegar

1 Pour the boiling water into a large bowl, so that is is about half full.

2 Add the vinegar, lemon juice and fresh mint leaves.

3 Hold your head over the bowl of water, with a towel draped over your head to keep the steam in.

4 Inhale for 10–15 minutes, stopping if the steam becomes uncomfortably hot.

Health tip
Try adding other ingredients such as fruit or herb vinegars with eucalyptus and cardamoms.

Sore throat gargle

Use this soothing gargle at the first sign of a sore throat. It can also be taken internally, 10ml/2 tsp at a time, 2–3 times a day. Use within a week.

INGREDIENTS
small handful each of fresh sage and
　thyme leaves
600ml/1 pint/2½ cups boiling water
30ml/2 tbsp cider vinegar
10ml/2 tsp honey
5ml/1 tsp cayenne pepper

1 Roughly chop the fresh sage and thyme leaves and place them in a large jug (pitcher).

2 Pour the boiling water over the herbs, cover and leave for 30 minutes.

3 Strain off the leaves and stir in the cider vinegar, honey and cayenne.

4 Gargle with a mouthful of the mixture to soothe a sore throat. Keep refrigerated for up to a week, but allow it to warm up to room temperature before using.

VINEGAR REMEDIES FOR FIRST AID

A useful cleanser and cooler, diluted or neat vinegar can be helpful for its antiseptic properties. Keep a small bottle with your first aid kit.

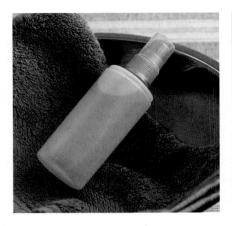

Sunburn

A vinegar and water solution will help to soothe burnt skin.

To treat a case of sunburn, soak a clean cloth in equal parts water and white distilled vinegar. Cover sunburnt areas with the cloth before going to bed. Leave on overnight if possible. Alternatively, put the vinegar and water mixture into a spray bottle and spray directly on to burnt skin.

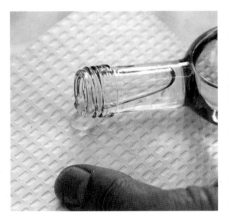

Burns

To treat minor burns, pour a little white distilled vinegar on to a paper towel and dab on to the affected area.

CAMPING TIP

Remember vinegar when picnicking or camping – in the absence of a formal first aid kit or antiseptic, vinegar is a useful cleanser for any minor scratches and cuts.

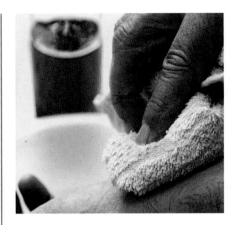

Cuts and grazes

Vinegar is a natural antiseptic. Making an antiseptic vinegar wipe for minor abrasions is less expensive and intrusive than harsh disinfectants.

Pour a small amount of cider vinegar on to a clean cotton wipe. Use to clean the skin around minor knocks and scrapes. It may sting a little, but it will help to prevent infection.

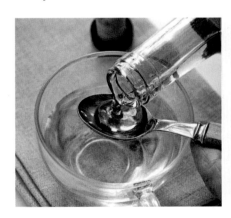

Hiccups

Drinking vinegar in water can halt an unfortunate attack of hiccups.

Add 5ml/1 tsp of cider vinegar to a glass of warm water. When suffering from hiccups, sip the mixture slowly and they will fade away.

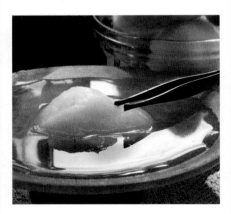

Cold sores

Use vinegar to soothe the pain and swelling of cold sores.

Soak a cotton wool ball in white distilled vinegar. Apply to the affected area two or three times a day.

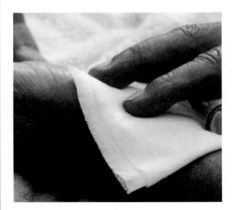

Bruises and swellings

Treat with a vinegar-soaked cloth.

Soak a cloth in equal parts white distilled vinegar and water. Wring out excess liquid. Apply to the bruise for at least 1 hour, holding in place with a bandage if necessary.

VINEGAR REMEDIES FOR CLEAR SKIN

A powerful astringent, a little cider vinegar diluted with spring water makes a zingy refresher or helpful potion to combat greasy skin.

Blocked pores

The alpha-hydroxy acids, or natural fruit acids, present in both strawberries and cider vinegar will act as a natural exfoliator when applied to the skin.

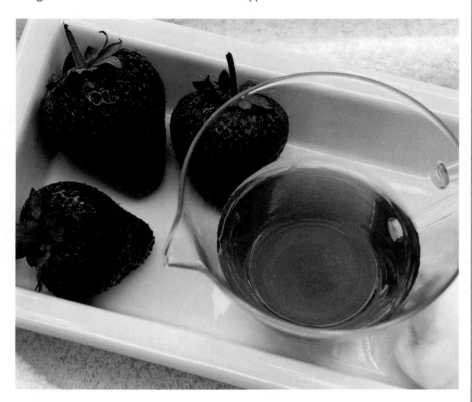

INGREDIENTS

3 large strawberries

55ml/¼ cup cider vinegar

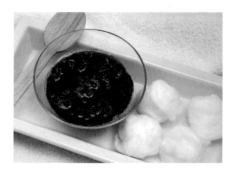

1 Remove the stalks from the strawberries, and in a small bowl, mash them. Add the cider vinegar, mixing well. Allow the mixture to stand for 2 hours, then strain into a bowl.

2 Apply the strawberry and vinegar mixture to the face with cotton wool and leave on the skin for as long as possible, preferably overnight.

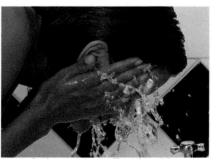

3 Wash the mixture off with cold water and a small amount of gentle cleanser if necessary. Your skin should feel soft and smooth.

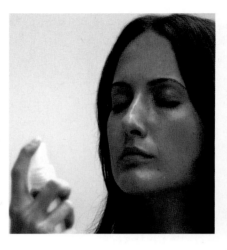

Acne

A gentle solution of cider vinegar and water can be used as an antiseptic face freshener.

Mix one part cider vinegar to 10 parts spring water. Transfer to a spray bottle, keep chilled and use as a face spritzer, making sure that the eyes are closed before spraying.

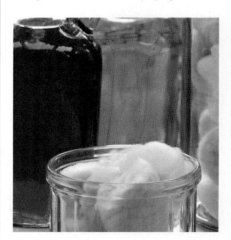

Chapped skin

Soothe cracked or chapped skin with cider vinegar.

Mix equal quantities of cider vinegar and spring water. Apply gently to the skin with a cotton wool ball.

VINEGAR REMEDIES FOR FOOTCARE

Feet are subject to daily pounding and are vulnerable to skin irritations. A little vinegar in a cool footbath makes a refreshing, cleansing footwash.

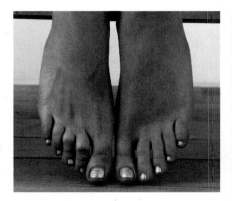

Dry or itchy skin

Soak in a vinegar bath to soften the skin on the feet, which is prone to dryness.

Add a few drops of cider vinegar to warm water. Soak the feet for 30 minutes to soothe dry or hard skin.

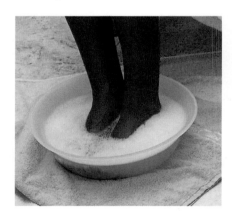

Corns

Traditionally, vinegar was applied as a bread poultice, by soaking bread in vinegar, then bandaging it on the corn. Now we know that corns need softening so that they can be gently rubbed off.

Soak the feet in warm soapy water and rub with olive oil to soften the corn. Rub off the corn with cotton wool. Use a dab of cider vinegar on a cotton wool ball to clean the area and prevent infection.

Athlete's foot

The cider vinegar in this foot bath helps to restore the pH balance of the skin, which becomes over-alkaline when suffering from this condition. Myrrh and tea-tree oil both have antifungal properties. If the condition is severe, with more than itching or with broken skin and blistering, it is important to follow medical advice. The ingredients can all be found at specialist health stores, or online.

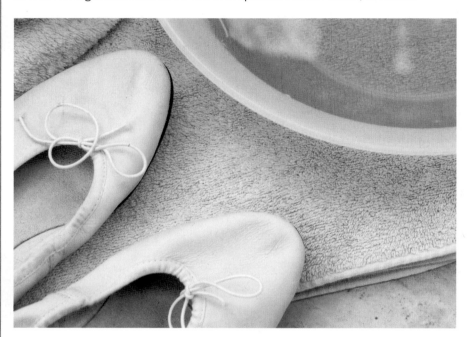

INGREDIENTS
25g/1oz dried sage
25g/1oz dried pot marigold flowers
1 large aloe vera leaf, chopped
15ml/1 tbsp myrrh granules
2.2 litres/4 pints/9 cups water
10 drops tea tree essential oil
60 ml/4 tbsp cider vinegar

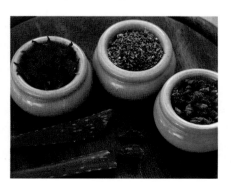

1 Pour the water into a pan and bring to the boil. Add the sage, dried pot marigold flowers, chopped aloe vera, and myrrh and cover. Allow to simmer for 20 minutes.

2 Allow the infusion to cool down a little, then strain into a large bowl.

3 Add the tea tree oil and vinegar to the bowl. Immerse the feet in the bowl for at least 15 minutes. Dry thoroughly.

TOENAIL FUNGUS

Drop a few drops of distilled white vinegar on the toenail three times a day to help clear up toenail fungus.

VINEGAR REMEDIES FOR HAIRCARE

Use vinegar in simple hair rinses, on its own or mixed with other ingredients, to promote general scalp health and to treat conditions such as dandruff, head lice and hair loss.

Dandruff rinse

Nasturtium is often used in hair products, and has a balancing effect on the skin. Use this hair rinse to soothe a dry, flaky scalp.

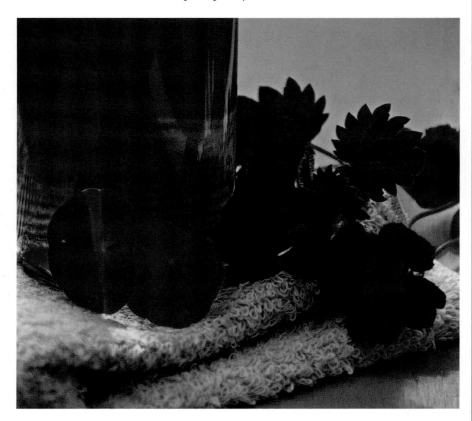

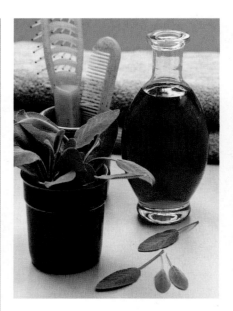

Hair loss

Vinegar is an excellent hair rinse for anyone and rinsing with cider vinegar may be helpful for those suffering from hair loss other than the genetic 'natural' balding experienced by men. An infusion of sage is also recommended – infuse sage leaves in a bottle of cider vinegar.

INGREDIENTS

25g/1oz nettle leaves

25g/1 oz nasturtium flowers and leaves

1 litre/1¾ pints/4 cups water

30ml/2 tbsp cider vinegar

30ml/2 tbsp witch hazel

1 Place the nettle leaves and nasturtium flowers and leaves in a large bowl.

2 Boil the water and pour it over the nettles and nasturtiums in the bowl. The nettle leaves will lose their sting in the boiling water.

3 Cover, allow to stand overnight, then strain off the leaves and flowers.

4 Add the cider vinegar and witch hazel to the strained liquid.

5 Pour through the hair as a final rinse every time you shampoo.

INGREDIENTS

50g/1oz fresh sage leaves

bottle of cider vinegar, about 600ml/1 pint/ 2½ cups

1 Pour enough of the vinegar out of the bottle to allow room for the sage leaves.

2 Wash and drain the sage leaves, then place them in the bottle of cider vinegar.

3 Leave for 2 weeks to infuse, then use as a hair rinse after washing.

HEAD LICE (NITS)

To treat an attack of headlice, first apply warmed vinegar to the scalp. Cover the head with a shower cap for 30 minutes, then rinse. Dip a fine-toothed nit comb in vinegar and comb through the hair to remove the lice and their eggs. Repeat the treatment for 3–5 days, until the lice have disappeared.

VINEGAR REMEDIES FOR INSECTS AND STINGS

As an emergency coolant, to cleanse and help reduce inflammation, and to keep them away, vinegar is useful for minor everyday insect attacks.

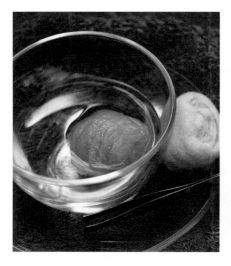

Insect bites
This will help to reduce any itching and irritation around the bite.

Soak a cotton wool ball in a small amount of white vinegar. Use this to clean the area around the insect bite.

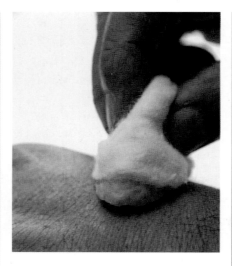

Jellyfish stings
Studies have shown that vinegar can deactivate the venom in jellyfish stings.

Dip a cotton wool ball in cider vinegar. Dab this on to the skin to reduce any pain and swelling. Seek medical attention.

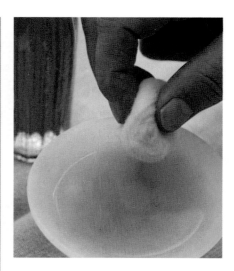

Wasp stings
This will work for bee stings too but remove the sting from the skin first.

Soak a cotton wool ball in cider vinegar. Apply directly to stings to alleviate pain and swelling.

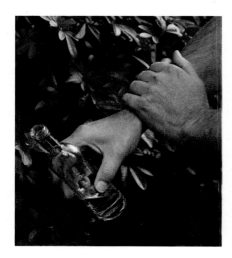

Insect repellent
Do not use a fruity sweetened vinegar as this may attract flies.

Pour a small amount of white vinegar into the palm of your hand. Rub the vinegar into the skin as a repellent.

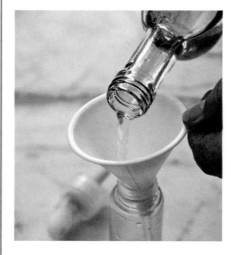

Bug spray
This natural bug spray is pet- and child-friendly.

Transfer a small amount of white vinegar to a spray bottle using a funnel. Use it as an economical bug spray.

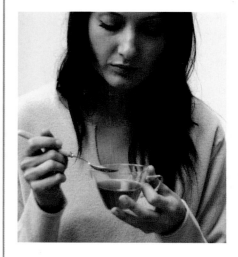

Mosquito repellent
Drink vinegar to keep mosquitoes away.

Drink 10ml/2 tsp cider vinegar a day to keep mosquitoes away. The vinegar is said to influence body odours – mosquitoes will find your perspiration unpleasant.

VINEGAR REMEDIES FOR MUSCULAR PROBLEMS

A refreshing vinegar bath soak will soothe tired or strained muscles, and will work wonders for the way you feel, aiding physical relaxation and calm.

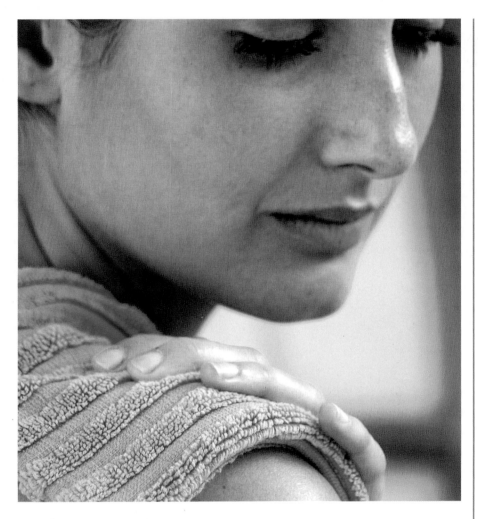

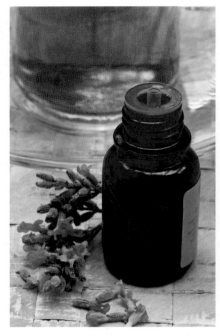

Muscle ache

Tired muscles can be soothed by relaxing in a hot bath scented with a combination of cider vinegar and lavender oil.

INGREDIENTS

15ml/1 tbsp cider vinegar

2–3 drops lavender oil

1 Fill a bath with warm water.

2 Add the cider vinegar and the lavender oil to the water to create a soothing bath.

Muscle compress

Soothe sore or aching muscles with a warm vinegar compress.

1 Mix 475ml/16fl oz/2 cups each of water and cider vinegar together in a large bowl.

2 Soak a small towel or flannel in the vinegar mixture.

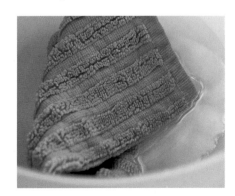

3 Heat the towel in the microwave for 20 seconds, until warm, then apply to the affected area.

MUSCLE TIREDNESS

A cider vinegar and honey drink is helpful for alleviating muscle tiredness after an exercise session. Put 5ml/1 tsp honey and 5ml/1 tsp cider vinegar in a cup and top up with hot water.

CRAMP

Vinegar is a traditional aid for relieving cramp, which can be caused by low levels of potassium. Take 5ml/1 tsp cider vinegar before going to bed to avoid waking up with cramp in the night.

VINEGAR REMEDIES FOR LATER LIFE

A little vinegar goes a long way to help combat some of the everyday symptoms of the long-standing conditions that can develop in later life.

Arthritis

Many people who suffer from arthritis swear by a daily dose of cider vinegar to help relieve the pain. Cherries are also commonly recommended to relieve the pain associated with arthritis and gout. Sufferers should make a batch of cherry cider vinegar to use as a dressing, in sauces or for drinks.

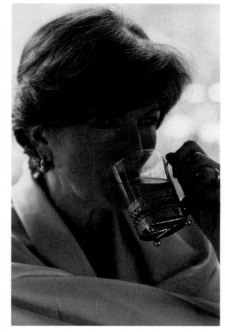

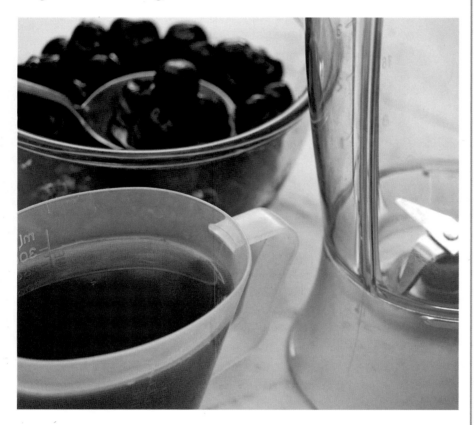

INGREDIENTS

450g/1 lb fresh or frozen cherries,
  stoned (pitted)
600ml/1 pint cider vinegar

1 Purée the fresh or frozen cherries in a blender with the cider vinegar.

2 Transfer to a bottle and store in the refrigerator. Shake well before using.

3 For a delicious drink, put 10ml/ 2 tsp cherry vinegar in a glass and top up with water.

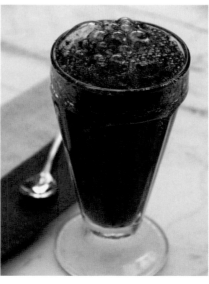

Stiff joints

If the body is short of potassium, joints can become stiff. Taking a teaspoon of cider vinegar in a glass of water will help replenish potassium levels.

Denture cleaning

Soak dentures in a glass of vinegar for up to an hour, for a natural alternative to your usual denture cleanser.

Bone health

Cider vinegar contains the elements manganese, magnesium, silicon and calcium, which can help with bone health. Either take a cider vinegar drink daily, or try cider vinegar supplements.

Age spots

Mix together the juice of an onion with an equal amount of vinegar and apply daily to age spots. After a few weeks you will notice the spots diminishing.

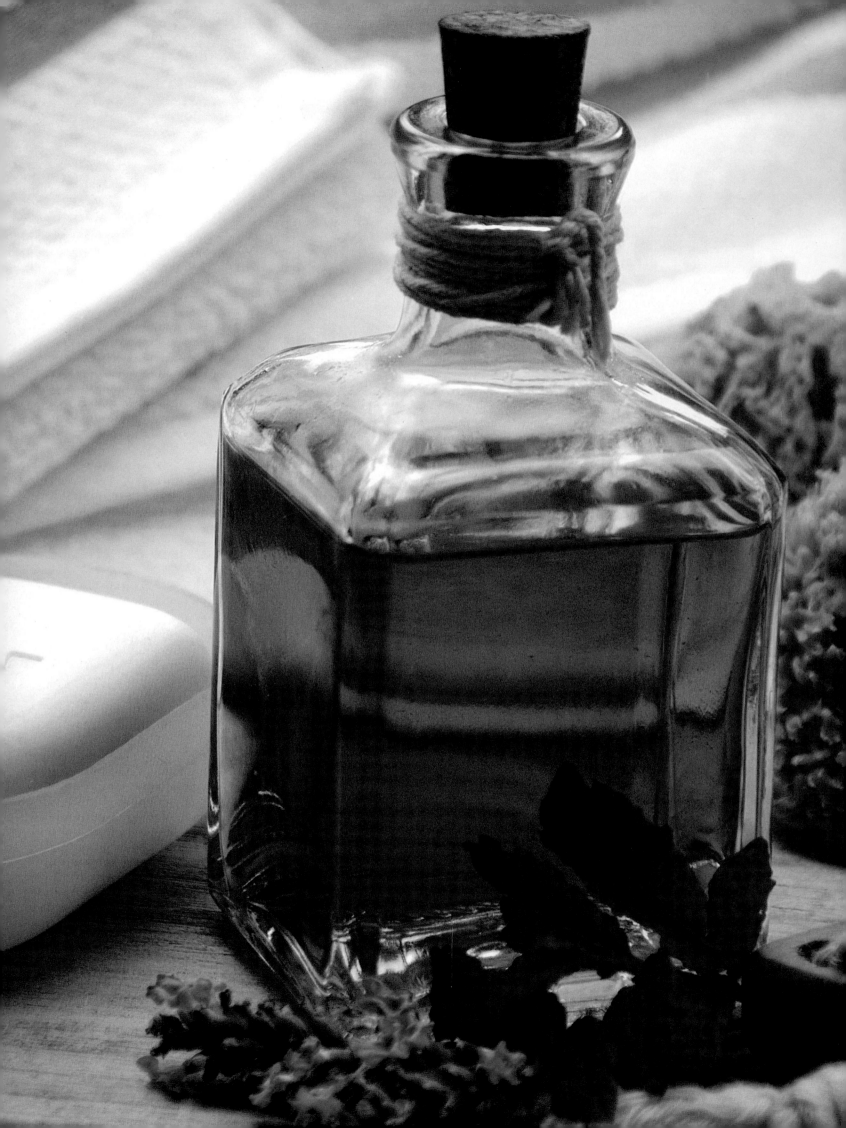

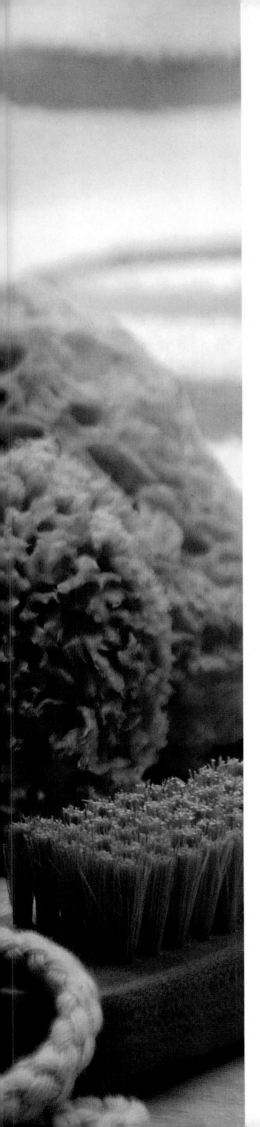

NATURAL BEAUTY WITH VINEGAR

This chapter shows how many home-made vinegar-based beauty treatments can be used instead of commercial products, with fabulous results. It is a natural exfoliator and astringent, and is a valuable addition to many skincare preparations. From head to toe, whether in hair rinses, bath soaks, face packs, body scrubs or foot baths, learn how to use vinegar in many simple potions that are superbly effective and pleasingly inexpensive.

Left: Cider vinegar is a great addition to the bathroom cabinet, and features in many home beauty treatments.

A TRADITIONAL BEAUTY INGREDIENT

Some of the most expensive and exotic beauty products rely on pure natural ingredients that can easily be combined at home with fantastic results.

Vinegar has been used in beauty treatments for thousands of years. Helen of Troy – reportedly the most beautiful woman in the world – bathed in vinegar to tone and condition her skin.

More recently, kitchen ingredients were frequently used in the boudoir before modern cosmetics became relatively inexpensive. As well as vinegar, olive oil, honey, rose water, witch hazel, oatmeal and milk were all typical ingredients used for cleaning and conditioning the hair and skin. Even after bought potions became more common, the majority of women were limited to just one pot of face cream. Pampering sessions involved creating natural concoctions at home from tips and recipes which had been passed down the generations from mother to daughter and between friends.

Deliciously uncomplicated

Discovering home-made beauty potions is great fun! Mixing and applying simple natural ingredients to the skin can be very satisfying. Many modern beauty treatments can be extremely harsh on the skin (as well as being expensive). Many types of face scrubs and peels can be too fierce for frequent use. Also, using many commercial products can result in a build-up of some substances that have to be removed by applying another; this is especially true for hair products.

WHICH VINEGAR TO USE?

Cider vinegar has a pleasant, slightly fruity odour that makes a positive contribution to beauty remedies.

Organic apple cider vinegars benefit from the goodness of the apples used as the basic ingredient. Cider vinegar is the best choice for facial treatments.

Distilled white vinegar is perfectly suitable for the majority of the remedies described here – it has a light refreshing smell.

Fruit vinegars are a good choice for beauty as long as they are not sweet or sweetened. Sweet vinegars are completely unsuitable and should not be used.

Malt, balsamic and red or white wine vinegars are also not suitable for use in beauty treatments.

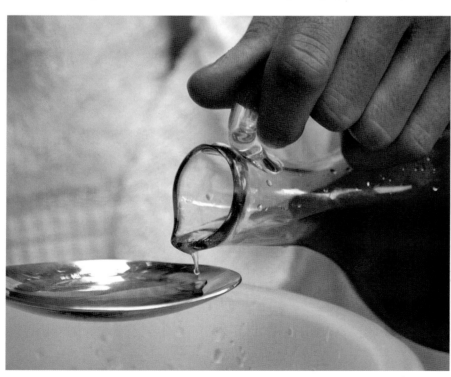

Above: Because cider vinegar is made from apples, it contains natural fruit acids, or alpha-hydroxy acids, which are very good for the skin, and are used in many cosmetics.

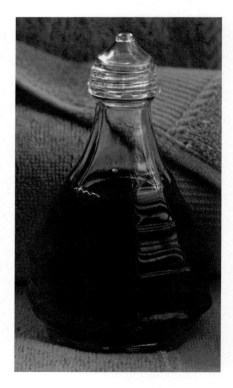

Above: Keep a bottle of cider vinegar handy on the bathroom shelf.

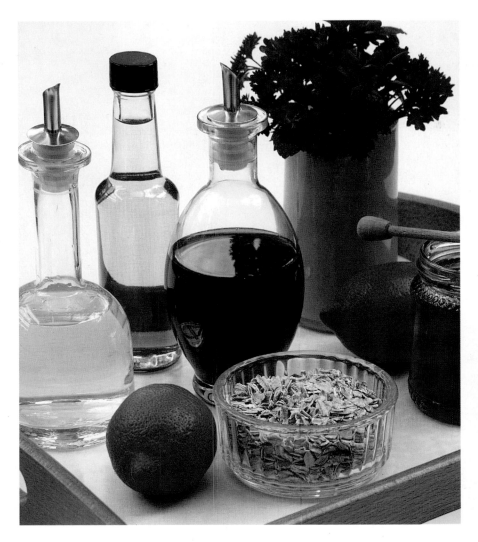

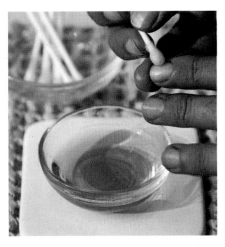

Above: Use a little vinegar as part of a natural manicure session.

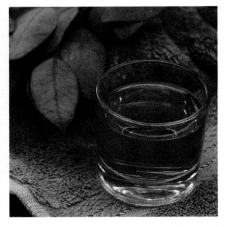

Above: Oils, herbs, fruit, honey and oats have long been prized alongside vinegar for their natural cleansing and conditioning properties.

Above: Vinegar can be used alone or with herbs to make fantastic hair treatments.

Making vinegar treatments

The vinegar treatments suggested here are all easy and inexpensive to prepare. They will help to bring a natural glow of health to hair, skin and nails without causing any damage. Home-made treatments containing cider vinegar will exfoliate and brighten the skin, due to the natural fruit acids, or alpha-hydroxy acids, in the vinegar.

Many soaps and cleansers are very alkaline, and the mild acidic qualities in vinegar will help to restore the natural pH balance of the skin. Use home-made vinegar treatments to complement favourite moisturizers and similar products.

There are many uses for vinegar in the bathroom. Add it to bath water for a refreshing soak, or use it in body washes or cleansers. Vinegar is famous for its ability to neutralize odours, and can even be used as a natural deodorant. Use vinegar to remove stains from the skin, or to prolong the life of nail varnish. It is a fantastic product to use on the hair, and can be used in conditioning rinses on its own or with herbs and herbal oils to remove product build-up.

The natural antibacterial qualities of vinegar make it particularly suitable to use in treatments for the feet, which can be prone to fungal infections. Make vinegar foot scrubs and foot washes to leave your feet refreshed. Use the natural exfoliating and brightening properties of cider vinegar in body scrubs, toners and face masks to leave your skin soft and smooth from top to toe.

ALPHA-HYDROXY ACIDS AND VINEGAR

Natural fruit acids, known as alpha-hydroxy acids (AHA), act as exfoliators by removing dead skin cells and stimulating production of replacements and natural moisturizers. These acids are found in different proportions and mixes in different fruit, including apples, citrus fruit, papaya, strawberries, grapes and pineapple. They are also present in cider vinegar, making it a great choice when preparing natural beauty treatments.

VINEGAR FOR BATHING AND CLEANSING

Adding a little refreshing vinegar to a warm bath is brilliant for restoring tired bodies and will help to balance the skin's natural pH balance.

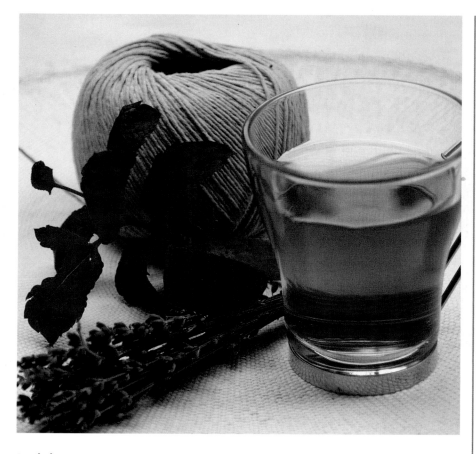

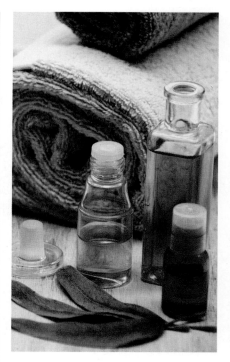

Bath bouquet

Using cider vinegar with herbs and orange will make a bath especially refreshing and relaxing.

INGREDIENTS
fresh mint, one bunch
fresh lavender, one bunch
rind of one orange
250ml/8fl oz/1 cup cider vinegar
baby oil
mild liquid bath soap

1 Tie the mint, lavender and orange rind together and place in the bath.

2 Pour the cup of cider vinegar into the bath on top of the bouquet.

3 Run a shallow layer of very hot water and leave to infuse for about 5 minutes.

4 Fill the bath with warm water to your preferred level, adding a few drops of baby oil and a mild liquid bath soap.

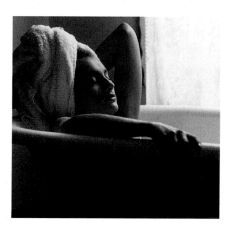

Head-clearing bath

Add a little cider vinegar, eucalyptus oil and tea tree oil to a hot bath for a head-clearing soak.

Scent neutralizer

To remove a scent that you have applied in error, or that has gone off, dab a little vinegar on to the skin that has been sprayed. The smell will be neutralized.

Deodorant

Using vinegar as a natural deodorant will not stop perspiration, but will neutralize body odour.

Cleanser

Most soap is alkaline, so using a mixture of equal parts vinegar to water helps to balance the skin's pH levels after bathing.

Exfoliating body wash

Vinegar is a natural exfoliator and this scrub is excellent for exfoliating arms and for encouraging circulation in the thighs and buttocks. It makes the skin all over smooth and moist. For a fabulous back scrub, enlist the help of a willing partner. Prepare a pad of towels and relax while someone gently scrubs and massages.

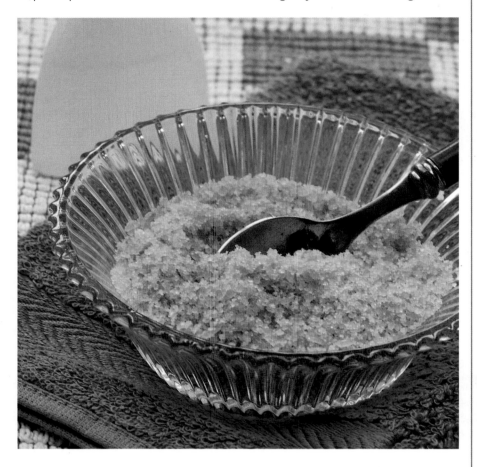

INGREDIENTS

1 small handful rice, uncooked

5ml/1 tsp white vinegar

2.5ml/½ tsp olive oil

10ml/2 tsp gentle body wash or shampoo

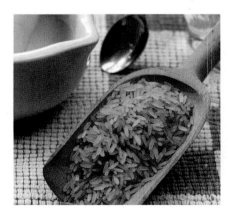

1 Crush the rice in a mortar with a pestle so that it has a gritty texture. Place in a bowl and mix in the vinegar.

2 Add the oil to the bowl. Stir in the body wash or shampoo to make a creamy mixture.

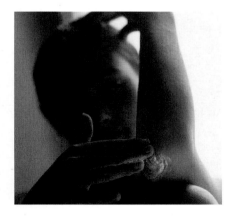

3 Shower with hot water and then scrub with the mixture, lathering it up to a foam. Concentrate on knees and elbows if there are any signs of rough skin.

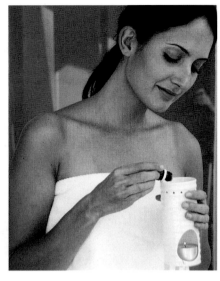

Bathroom aroma

A candle burner for heating aromatic oil in water is ideal for creating a relaxing environment for soaking in the bath. For a refreshing aroma, add a little white vinegar to the water – about 1.25ml/¼ teaspoon – as well as a few drops of oil.

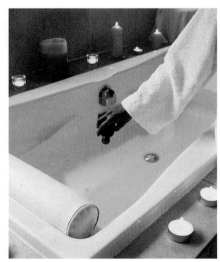

Refreshing bath

Pour some cider vinegar into the bath for a refreshing soak. This will also help to prevent mild bacterial and fungal infections.

Aftershave

A mixture of equal parts cider vinegar to water will work as an aftershave. The acetic acid in the vinegar acts as an antiseptic on cuts or abrasions.

VINEGAR FOR HAND TREATMENTS

A valuable cleanser and antiseptic, vinegar can be used to remove stains from the hands, to prepare fingernails for varnish and to prevent infection.

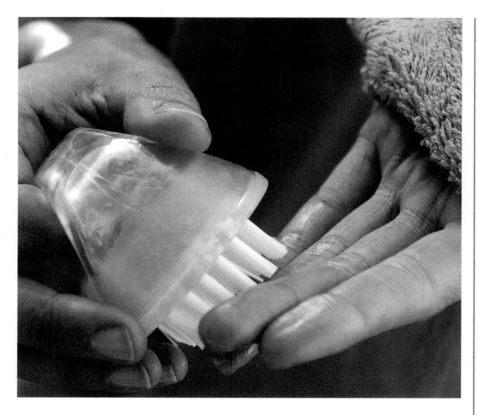

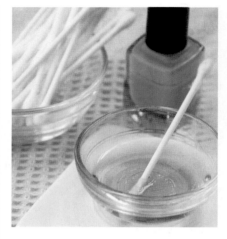

Longer lasting nail varnish

Apply vinegar underneath varnish to make it last longer before chipping.

Dip a cotton bud in vinegar. Use to clean the surface of the fingernail before applying a base coat or nail varnish.

Stain remover

This is a good way of removing fruit stains from the hands, for example after picking blackberries or strawberries. Margarine or lard and granulated (white) sugar make an excellent scouring agent for removing stubborn stains from hands when used with vinegar.

INGREDIENTS

45ml/2 tbsp vinegar
30ml/2 tbsp granulated (white) sugar
45ml/2 tbsp margarine or lard
a bowl of hot soapy water
vegetable oil

1 Prepare a small saucer each of vinegar, margarine or lard and granulated sugar.

2 Rub in the vinegar with a nail brush.

3 Scrub the hands with the fat and then finally the granulated sugar.

4 Repeat if necessary until the staining comes away, then wash in hot soapy water. Dry and massage with a little vegetable oil.

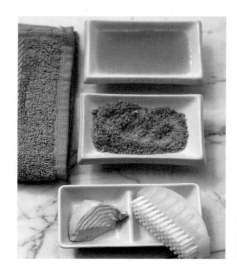

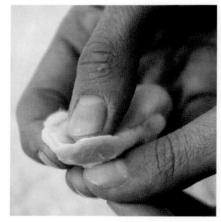

Hand health

When they are frequently in and out of water, hands are prone to fungal infection under and around the nail area. Use vinegar to prevent this.

Use a cotton wool ball dipped in vinegar to clean around and under the nail area. Dry under a hot air drier or shake the hands dry.

VINEGAR FOR HAIRCARE

Using vinegar in a hair rinse is a brilliant way to achieve super-shiny hair. It can also be used to lighten the hair or on dyed hair to keep colour strong and fresh.

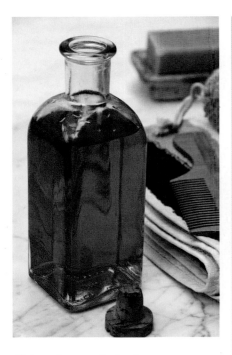

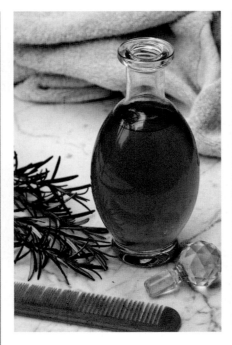

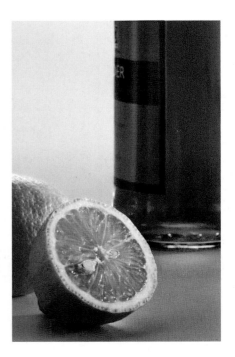

Cider vinegar hair rinse

This gentle vinegar rinse will remove the build-up caused by using products such as hairsprays and waxes on the hair.

INGREDIENTS
washing up liquid
250ml/18 fl oz/1 cup cider vinegar
1 litre/1¾ pints/4 cups warm water

1 First use a little mild washing up liquid to shampoo the hair, massaging the scalp gently. Try to avoid rubbing the hair up into a tangle. Comb through any tangles with your fingers.

2 Repeat and then rinse the soap from the hair completely.

3 Put the cider vinegar into a suitable bottle, add the warm water and then use the mixture as the final hair rinse for shiny, healthy-looking hair.

Rosemary hair rinse

Use a vinegar rinse once a week to improve the health of your hair. Rosemary is a good conditioner for dark hair.

INGREDIENTS
50g/2oz sprigs of rosemary
250ml/18 fl oz/1 cup cider vinegar
10 drops rosemary oil

1 Infuse the rosemary sprigs in enough boiling water to cover them, for 12 hours.

2 Strain, add the vinegar and rosemary oil, then pour into a bottle to use as required.

CLEAN HAIR TONGS

If you notice a build-up of hair products on curling tongs or straightening irons, they can be cleaned with a vinegar solution. Mix equal parts water and vinegar with a pinch of salt.

Natural hair lightener

Lemon juice is known for its lightening effect on the hair. The acid in the vinegar will help to accelerate the process.

INGREDIENTS
juice of two lemons
120ml/4fl oz/½ cup cider vinegar

1 Mix the lemon juice and vinegar in a spray bottle. For subtle highlights, separate strands of hair and spray with the mixture, or spray hair all over.

2 Leave for 10 minutes then wash off.

COLOUR FIXER

When hair has been coloured with a natural product such as henna, use vinegar as a colour fixer. Once the henna has been washed out, apply 120ml/4fl oz/½ cup vinegar, massage into the hair and rinse.

VINEGAR FOR FOOTCARE

Inexpensive cider vinegar is ideal for everyday footcare – keep a small bottle in the bathroom cupboard and use these treatments regularly for softer skin.

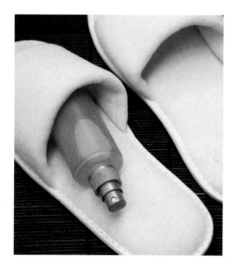

Refreshing spritzer

Make a vinegar spritzer to cool tired feet and legs.

INGREDIENTS

rosewater

cider vinegar

a few drops of eucalyptus oil

1 In a small, fine sprayer, mix 6 parts rosewater with 1 part vinegar and add the eucalyptus oil.

2 Shake well and place in the refrigerator to chill for at least an hour.

3 Spray lightly on tired feet and legs, then put the feet up while sipping a refreshing cider vinegar and herb or fruit tea.

TOENAIL CARE

Use a cotton bud dipped in vinegar to clean around toenails after trimming, filing, tidying and buffing. Then massage in oil, lotion or foot cream.

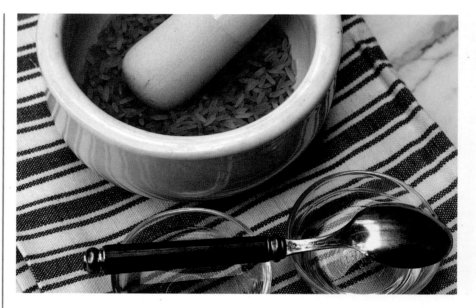

Rough skin scrub

Mix vinegar with crushed rice and oil to make a scrub which will leave your feet smooth and soft.

INGREDIENTS

1 handful rice, uncooked

5ml/1 tsp cider vinegar

2.5 ml/½ tsp oil

1 Crush the rice using a pestle and mortar to a gritty texture. Place in a bowl and mix in the vinegar until well combined, then add 2.5 ml/½ tsp oil. This makes enough for two foot scrubbing sessions. Keep the excess in a covered pot in the refrigerator for up to a week or freeze it.

2 Prepare a bowl of hot water for washing the feet after scrubbing and a small towel or clean dish towel on which to scrub them (this saves getting the scrub in the bottom of the bath).

3 Wash the feet in hot soapy water to soften the skin, then pat them dry. Place on the towel.

4 Take a spoonful of rice scrub in the palm of one hand and rub it into the foot, then use both hands to scrub the skin, working around the edges of the soles and toes as well as the heels to remove rough skin gently. Rinse well, then dry thoroughly.

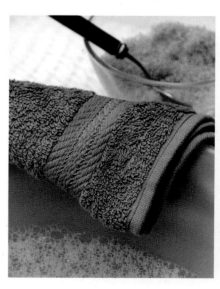

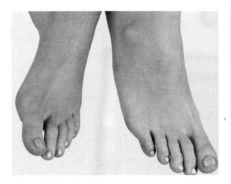

Soothing wax pack

This brightens and softens the skin as well as conditioning the nails.

INGREDIENTS

paraffin wax or nail or hand treatment wax, enough to cover both feet

vinegar, for massaging

2 pieces of clear film (plastic wrap), about 30x40cm

olive oil

1 Place each piece of clear film on a separate large folded towel.

2 Melt the paraffin wax or nail or hand treatment wax according to packet instructions in a large bowl over a pan of hot water. The bowl should be large enough for the toes to be placed in it.

3 Massage vinegar into one foot, working it well between the toes and around the nails. Check the temperature of the melted wax – it must be hot but not hot enough to be uncomfortable or burn the skin. Place as much of the foot as possible in the bowl and spoon the wax over it.

4 When the foot is coated in wax, place it on a piece of cling film. Spoon a little wax over any bare patches. Fold the cling film around the foot and then wrap the foot in the towel.

5 Repeat with the other foot. Relax for 30 minutes. Unwrap the feet and remove the wax. Massage with olive oil to finish.

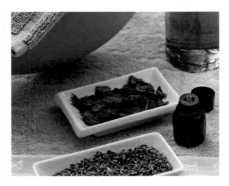

Lavender and vinegar foot bath

Soothe worn-out feet with vinegar, relaxing lavender and lemon verbena.

INGREDIENTS

15g/½oz dried lemon verbena

30ml/2 tbsp dried lavender

5 drops lavender essential oil

30ml/2 tbsp cider vinegar

1 Put the lemon verbena and lavender in a basin and pour in enough hot water to cover the feet.

2 When it has cooled add the lavender oil and cider vinegar.

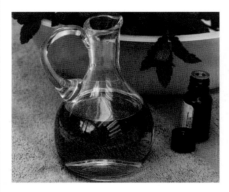

Footwash

Relax tired feet with vinegar and mint.

INGREDIENTS

12–15 mint leaves, crushed

3–4 drops tea tree oil

vinegar

1 Add the mint, tea tree oil and a little vinegar to a bowl of hot water.

2 Soak feet for 15 minutes.

FOOTCARE TIPS

• Washing in warm water with vinegar added is an old-fashioned treatment for all sorts of foot complaints, from corns to smelly feet. Vinegar deters fungal and bacterial activity, which is why it can help to prevent odours and foot infections. On its own it is not necessarily enough to cure these type of problems but it is a useful preventative lotion, for example to wipe out trainers and for cleansing feet immediately after using public swimming pools and showers.

• Walking barefoot in changing rooms is enough to pick up unwanted infection, so it is a good idea to wear flip-flops and wipe them over with a little vinegar when they are dry.

• As well as using vinegar in a footwash, a persistent problem of foot odour can be treated by rubbing a little vinegar over the feet after washing and drying every morning and night.

• Socks, tights or stockings should ideally be cotton and they should be washed daily. Remove them at the end of the working day, then wash and dry the feet before rubbing lightly with vinegar. Then leave the feet to air for the evening, if possible, rather than wearing socks or slippers.

• Keep footwear clean and allow it to air. Avoid plastics and materials that do not allow air to pass into the shoes and sweat to evaporate. Use suitable insoles that can be replaced or washed frequently. Sprays to prevent micro-organisms from infecting footwear can be expensive, especially for everyday use. Instead, wipe out shoes with a cotton pad dipped in vinegar and leave to air and dry every day.

• Try to avoid wearing the same pair of shoes too often. After sport, always remove training shoes from sports bags and allow them to air.

VINEGAR FOR SOFT SKIN

A cornucopia of natural oils, herbs and other gentle ingredients can be mixed with cider vinegar to make these fabulous skincare potions.

Refreshing hot cloth

This is a good pore-opening process that works very well before using a face scrub or applying a face pack. Eucalyptus oil has a lovely fresh smell.

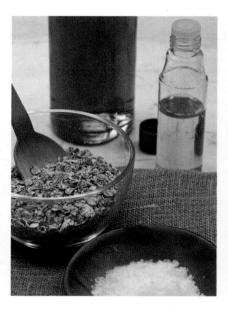

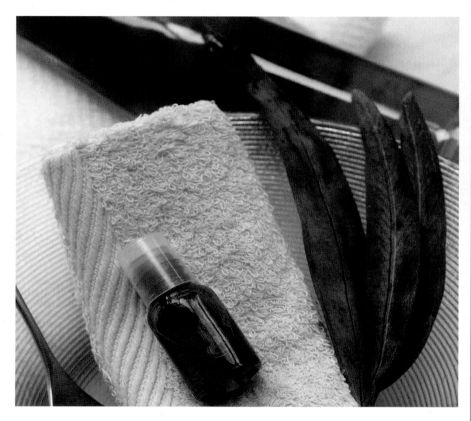

INGREDIENTS

15 ml/1 tbsp cider vinegar

a few drops of eucalyptus oil

1 Add the cider vinegar and eucalyptus oil to a small bowl of boiling water. Place a clean face cloth in the bowl and swirl it around.

2 Remove any make-up and wash with hot water, then dry the face.

3 Drain the hot cloth and wring it out, leaving it moist but not wet. Take care not to burn the hands and be sure that the cloth is not too hot for the face.

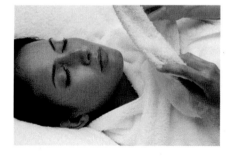

4 Lay the cloth over the face, pressing it gently around the nose, chin and forehead. Lie back and relax for a few minutes while the cloth is hot.

5 When the cloth cools, remove it and apply a face pack or scrub while the pores are open.

Oatmeal salt scrub

Exfoliating vinegar is mixed with moisturizing oil, salt and oatmeal.

INGREDIENTS

30 ml/2 tsp fine oatmeal

30 ml/2 tsp salt

2.5 ml/½ tsp sweet almond oil or
   avocado oil

2.5 ml/½ tsp cider vinegar

1 Mix the fine oatmeal with the salt and sweet almond oil or avocado oil in a bowl. When thoroughly combined, stir in the cider vinegar.

3 Wash the face with hot water and mild soap, then pat dry, leaving the skin moist.

4 Gently exfoliate with the scrub, working around the nose and chin, up the cheeks and across the forehead. Avoid the delicate areas around the eyes.

5 Rinse well with hot water and pat dry.

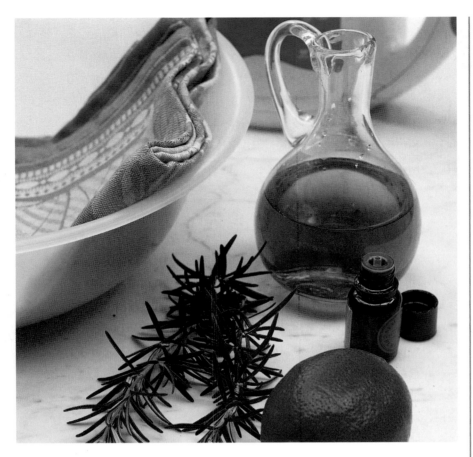

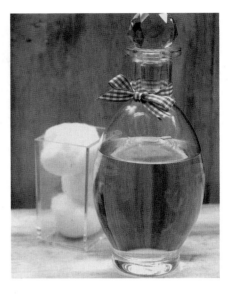

Face steaming

This is a great way of opening the pores and drawing out dirt and oils. It is good before applying a deep cleansing mask, such as a mud mask.

INGREDIENTS

15 ml/1 tbsp cider vinegar

a few drops of lavender or tea tree oil

a sprig of fresh herb such as rosemary
 or mint

rind of 1 lemon or lime

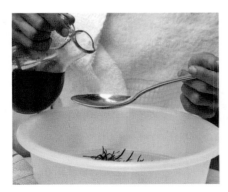

1 Prepare a large bowl of boiling water and add the vinegar. Add your chosen essential oil and/or herbs.

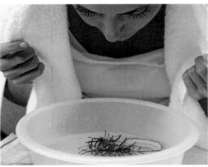

2 Hold your face over the steaming bowl and drape a towel over both head and bowl. Your pores should be open and the face sweating profusely. Steam your face for 5–10 minutes, but stop if it becomes at all uncomfortable.

STEAMING TIPS

If you are unused to steaming your face take care not to have your face too close to the water. Lower your face slowly while pulling over the towel to make sure the steam is not too fierce. Electric face steamers are inexpensive and great for regular cleansing. Add a little cider vinegar to the water.

Rose petal toner

Infusions of flowers make excellent toners.

INGREDIENTS

40g/1½oz fresh rose petals

600ml/1 pint/2½ cups boiling water

15ml/1 tbsp cider vinegar

1 Put the rose petals in a bowl, pour over the boiling water and add the vinegar. Cover and leave to stand for 2 hours, then strain into a clean bottle.

2 Apply with cotton wool (cotton balls) after removing make-up. Keep chilled and used up within a few days as this will soon deteriorate.

Vinegar and rosewater freshener

Use this freshener around oily areas, such as the nose and chin. Avoid the area around the eyes.

INGREDIENTS

cider vinegar

rosewater

1 Mix 1 part cider vinegar with 3 parts rosewater and pour into a small bottle.

2 To use, dampen a cotton ball and then apply a little of the mix, then pat it over the skin to close the pores after cleansing.

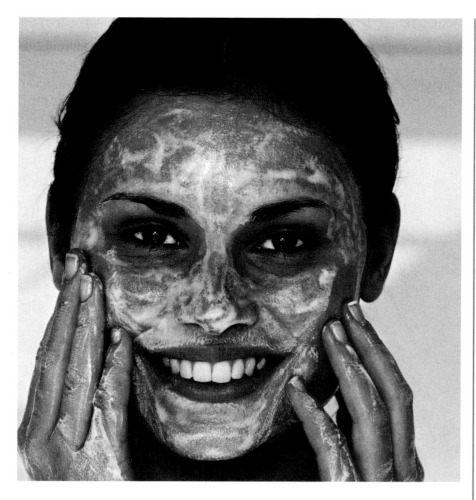

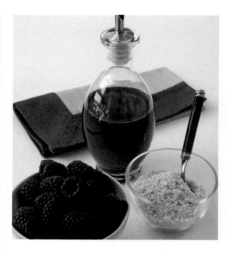

Almond and raspberry face pack

This vinegar mixture will brighten skin.

INGREDIENTS

30ml/2 tbsp ground almonds

5ml/1 tsp unsweetened raspberry vinegar

Place the ground almonds in a bowl, add the unsweetened raspberry vinegar and mix well. Spread over the face using your fingertips. Leave for 30 minutes before rinsing.

Egg white face pack

The protein in egg whites can do wonders for the skin, particularly when mixed with cider vinegar and oil.

INGREDIENTS

1 egg white

5 ml/1 tsp cider vinegar

2.5 ml/¹/₂ tsp sweet almond or avocado oil

30 ml/2 tbsp cornflour (cornstarch)

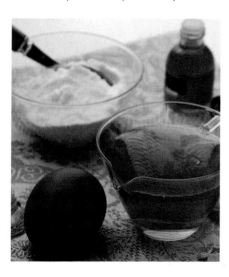

1 Break up the egg white with a fork, then stir in the cider vinegar and sweet almond or avocado oil.

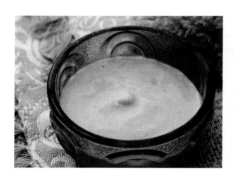

2 Add the cornflour (cornstarch) and stir it in well to give a creamy mixture.

3 Wash and dry your face, then spread the pack smoothly over the skin.

4 Lie down somewhere quiet and relax for about 30 minutes.

5 Rinse off the pack with warm water before moisturizing.

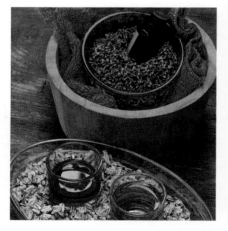

Brightening oat face pack

Combine moisturizing oil with vinegar.

INGREDIENTS

30ml/2 tbsp rolled oats

5ml/1 tsp cider vinegar

5ml/1 tsp olive oil

3 drops of lavender oil

Mix the oats with the cider vinegar and olive oil. Add the lavender oil and spread over the face, avoiding the eyes. Rinse after 30 minutes.

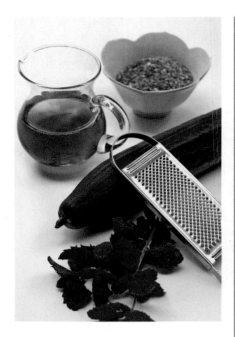

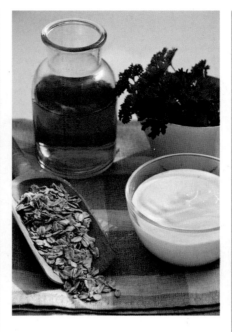

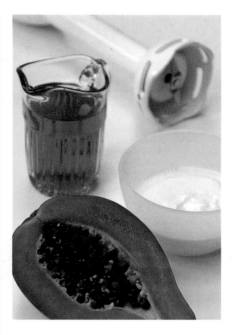

Cucumber and mint face pack

Use the natural cooling and cleansing properties of cucumber with cider vinegar to make a refreshing face pack.

INGREDIENTS

cucumber, about 2.5cm/1 in length

fresh mint leaves

2.5ml/½ tsp cider vinegar

15ml/1 tbsp fine oatmeal

1 Wash and finely grate the cucumber (skin and all) into a small bowl.

2 Add a few chopped fresh mint leaves and mix in the cider vinegar. Stir in the fine oatmeal and spread the mixture over the face.

3 Chill out for 15 – 30 minutes before rinsing with lukewarm water and spritzing with chilled spring water.

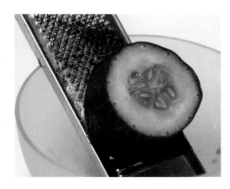

Vinegar, parsley and yogurt pack

Parsley and cider vinegar are both known for their astringent qualities. This soothing mask is great for oily skin.

INGREDIENTS

a handful of fresh parsley

5ml/1 tsp cider vinegar

15ml/1 tbsp rolled oats

30ml/2 tbsp low-fat yogurt

1 Finely chop the fresh parsley and place it in a small bowl. Add the vinegar and mix well.

2 Stir in the rolled oats until thoroughly combined, then gently mix in the low-fat yogurt.

3 Spread this all over the face, avoiding the eyes. Relax for 15 minutes before washing it off.

ENLARGED PORES

Mix 30ml/2 tbsp almond flour with enough water to make a paste. Apply evenly to the face, paying particular attention to areas with enlarged pores. Leave for for 20 minutes. Rinse with warm water, then apply a solution of apple cider vinegar and water.

Stimulating fruit paste

Papaya contains alpha-hydroxy acids, (also present in the vinegar), which have an exfoliating effect on the skin.

INGREDIENTS

fresh papaya

15ml/1 tbsp cider vinegar

15ml/1 tbsp plain low-fat yogurt

1 Peel and deseed the papaya. Cut two slices about 1cm/½ inch thick.

2 Dice the flesh of the two papaya slices and place in a food processor or blender.

3 Add the cider vinegar and yogurt and blend to make a smooth paste.

4 Cleanse the skin as usual, then apply the fruit paste evenly to the face, taking care to avoid the delicate skin around the eyes.

5 Leave for about 20 minutes, then rinse off with warm water.

Beauty tip

If papaya is difficult to get hold of, you can use other fresh fruits such as pineapple, peach, strawberries or grapes.

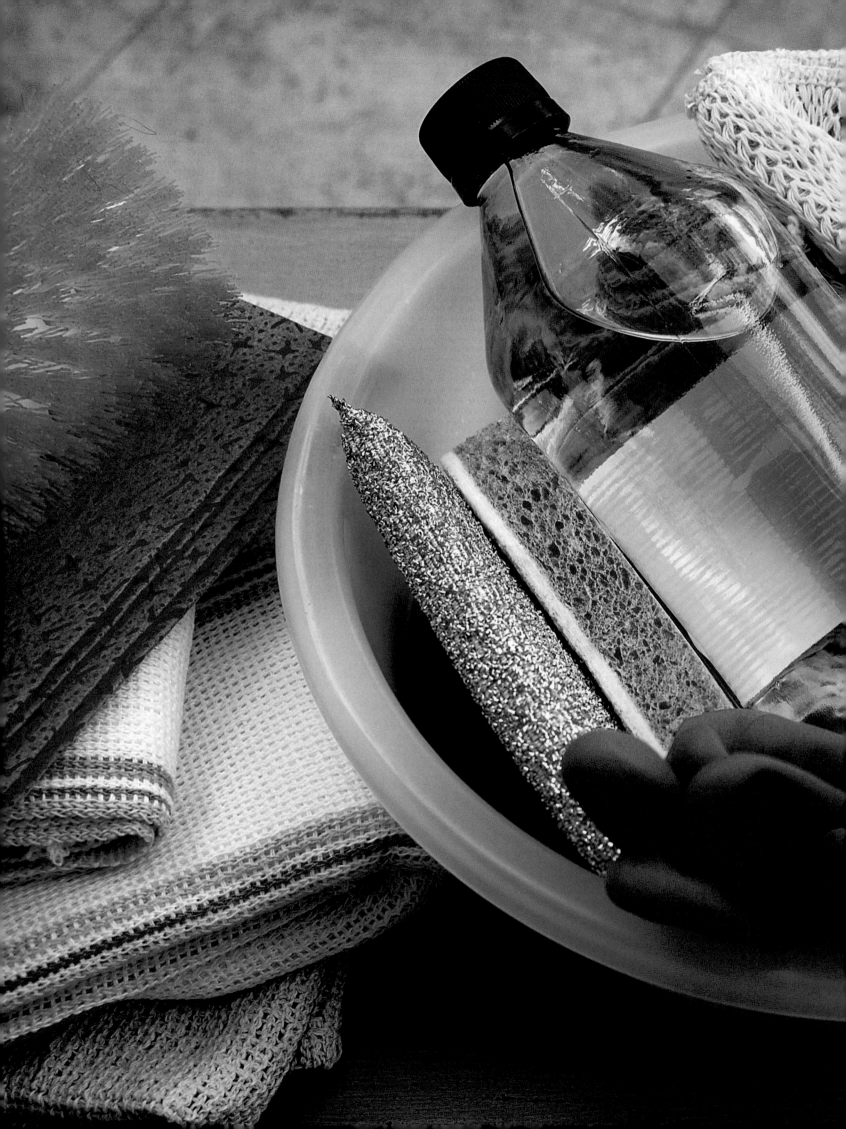

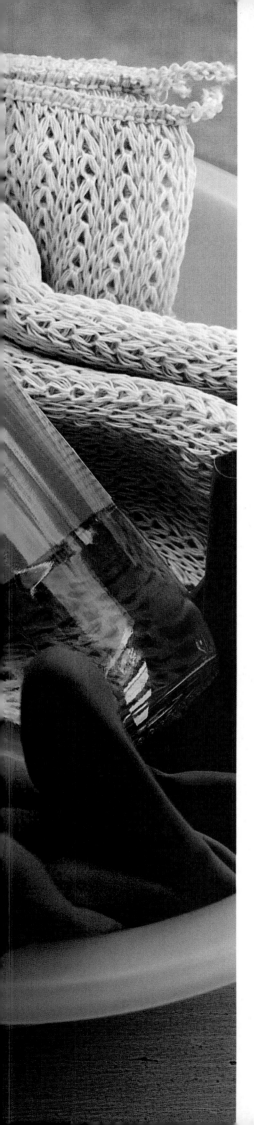

VINEGAR IN THE HOME AND GARDEN

Walls and windows, floors and furniture can all sparkle with the aid of a little vinegar. Inside and outside, this chapter includes all sorts of suggestions for effective vinegar alternatives to costly commercial cleaning products, from polishing mirrors, cleaning paintwork, and removing stains to deodorizing rooms, trapping insects and killing weeds. There are ideas for laundry, car valeting, home decorating and gardening, as well as using vinegar to help ensure pets are in peak condition.

Left: Once you start using vinegar instead of chemical cleaning products you will be amazed at its effectiveness.

VINEGAR AROUND THE HOME

Vinegar brings a sparkle as well as a fresh aroma to many everyday cleaning tasks, from refreshing the refrigerator to making windows gleam.

Vinegar has a great variety of traditional uses as a household cleaner. It can be used for minor everyday tasks as well as renovation and restoration projects. It is a traditional stain remover for laundry as well as a type of 'rinse aid' for shiny surfaces that are to be polished off with a clean dry cloth. It is also useful for removing built-up polishes and grime found on old wooden furniture and fittings.

Discovering vinegar as a cleaner and restorer is exciting because it is neither as noxious nor expensive as many of the harsh commercial products can be.

As many household uses for vinegar were established generations before modern fabrics and furnishings were even invented, many of the methods are particularly useful for treating old and antique items, such as furniture or even old linens that can easily be damaged by modern detergents or bleaches.

Cleaning power

Vinegar is also useful for cleaning modern materials and surfaces. It is less harsh and less expensive than the majority of cleaning products and ideal for everyday use, especially to prevent a build-up of dirt, such as scale or grease in sinks, wash basins and drains.

Vinegar is great for cleaning glass, leaving it sparkling and free from greasy smearing. As well as windows, mirrors and items of glassware, try vinegar for glass splash-backs, doors and surfaces in the kitchen and bathroom. It is also excellent for polishing many modern

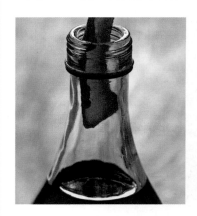

SCENTED VINEGAR

Add lavender or mint sprigs and strips of lemon rind to a bottle of distilled malt vinegar that is to be used for cleaning to give a fresh aroma.

metal finishes, including stainless steel and chrome, shiny rigid plastic surfaces and paintwork. It can be used to clean appliances such as irons, dishwashers, kettles and coffee-makers.

Vinegar may be used in the first stage of cleaning, for example to wipe off greasy stains from a surface, or as a final polish after washing down with hot soapy water. Vinegar can be added to the final rinsing water after washing. Alternatively, when the surface is washed and completely dried, vinegar can be applied as a polish by using it on a clean lint-free cloth. Vinegar can be used in the garden for cleaning or restoring furniture, as well as an insect and cat repellent.

General preparation

It is easy to forget that vinegar is an acid, and can damage as well as clean, so before launching in with bottle and cloth or brush, take a few moments to check

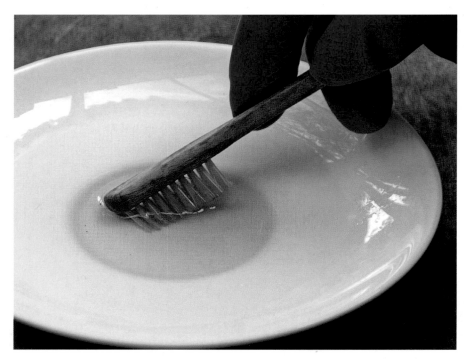

Above: Vinegar is particularly suitable for use on antique wooden furniture, but it should always be tested on a small out-of-sight area first.

WHICH VINEGAR TO USE?

Malt vinegar is the most economical choice for household and garden use as it can be purchased in large quantities and is less expensive than wine or cider vinegars. Distilled white vinegar is clear and therefore better than dark vinegar, which may stain fabrics. However, when cleaning extremely dirty old wood or tarnished metal, ordinary malt vinegar does just as well, especially in the first stages.

Similarly, for garden and outdoor use, inexpensive malt vinegar is the most sensible choice, if there is no danger of staining. Before cleaning new items, fabrics or surfaces with vinegar, always read the manufacturer's instructions to check that using vinegar (a mild acid) will not cause any damage.

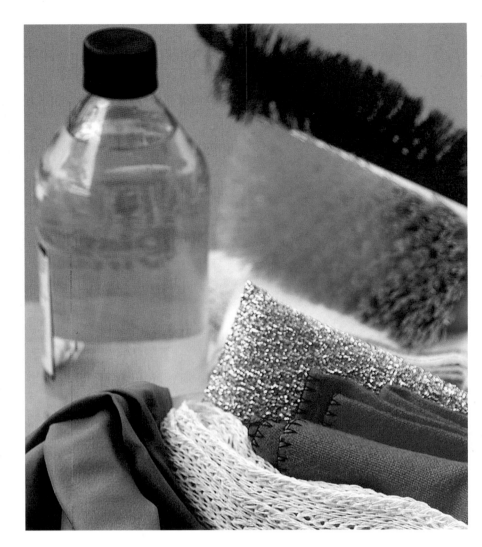

Above: Storing a bottle of vinegar in the cupboard with other cleaning products and materials will help you get into the habit of using it around the house.

the effect vinegar may have on the item and to protect the surrounding area. Begin by reading the manufacturer's instructions for a particular item.

Always experiment on a small area of fabric, furniture or material that is hidden or, preferably, separate from the item to be treated to make sure that the solution used will not cause any adverse reaction or damage.

Ensure that surrounding areas are covered or protected in some way, or that the items to be cleaned or restored are removed. For example, door fittings, such as handles, should be removed if they are to be restored to avoid damaging surrounding wood. Paintwork or frames around mirrors or glass should be protected by applying a suitable masking tape; conversely, when cleaning frames, it is important to avoid damaging mirrors, glass or the contents of a frame.

Gather together everything required before starting work. This is particularly practical for cleaning, rinsing, drying and polishing with efficiency when speed is important.

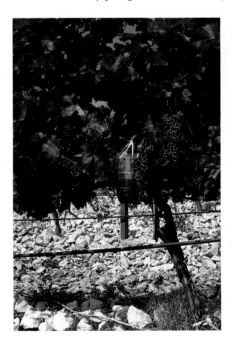

Above: A mixture of vinegar and fruit juice is used to attract flies away from grapes.

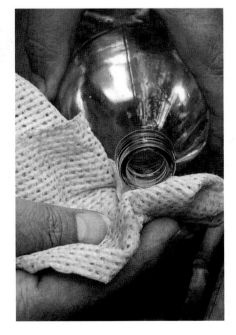

Above: Distilled white vinegar can be used to clean resilient surfaces.

VINEGAR FOR FURNITURE, FRAMES AND MIRRORS

Vinegar has a long history of use by professional polishers and restorers on wooden furniture – it is good for gentle renovation rather than harsh stripping.

Wooden furniture

Vinegar and oils are traditional cleaning and restoring agents for old wood. A paint brush, toothbrush or special curved furniture brush are useful for getting into awkward corners or cleaning moulding and joinery.

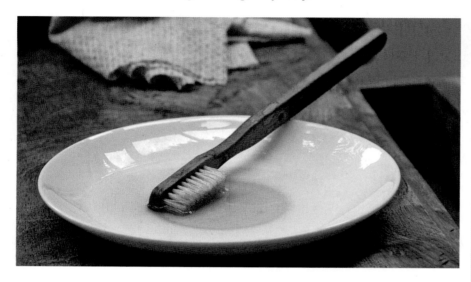

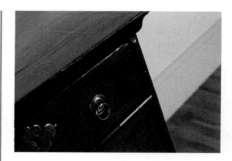

Mahogany bloom

Polished mahogany furniture sometimes develops a bloom or 'misty' surface, which can be prevented with vinegar.

INGREDIENTS
15ml/1 tbsp vinegar
5ml/1 tsp linseed oil
5ml/1 tsp turpentine

INGREDIENTS
60ml/4tbsp vinegar
wax polish or furniture oil

1 Pour the vinegar into a dish and dampen a brush or small piece of wire wool, then rub a small hidden area of the item.

2 Wipe with a damp cloth and then with a dry cloth. Check the result – depending on the finish and the extent of cleaning required, a quick rub and polish will remove a light build-up of old polish and dirt.

3 When a small patch has been cleaned successfully, begin to work all over the item. Clean small areas at a time, being consistent, and drying them well. Change the vinegar and wire wool frequently.

FURNITURE TIPS

Wear rubber gloves to avoid staining the hands and nails. Always work with the grain of the wood, rubbing along it, not against it. Use light pressure and repeat the process rather than being too fierce with one application.

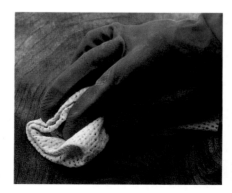

4 When the item is clean, give it a rub over with a damp cloth moistened with vinegar. Quickly dry it before buffing to a polish with a suitable oil or wax polish.

1 Prepare two solutions: in one bowl add the vinegar to 120ml/4 fl oz/½ cup hot water. In another bowl, mix the linseed oil and turpentine with 600 ml/1 pint/2½ cups water.

2 Wring out a cloth in the hot water and vinegar and wipe the wood. Follow with a cloth wrung out in the oil and turpentine solution. Polish with a chamois leather to dry the wood and give it a shine.

3 Repeat if necessary. Wipe down with vinegar water occasionally to prevent a build-up of bloom.

REMOVING RINGS

If wet drinks glasses have left rings on wooden furniture, remove them by rubbing with a mixture of one part olive oil, one part white distilled vinegar.

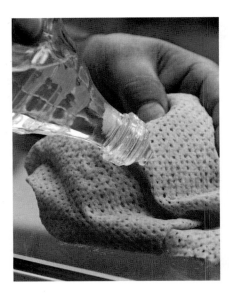

Glass tabletops

Rub glass surfaces with a vinegar cloth to remove any smears and greasy marks.

Wash the tabletop or surface as usual with soapy water and dry with a clean dish towel. Then dampen a clean cloth and sprinkle a little vinegar over it. Rub the surface with the vinegar cloth then polish it again with a clean dry cloth.

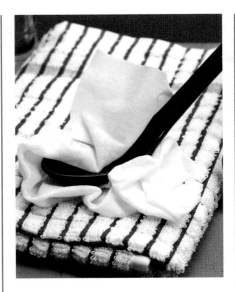

Lacquer

Bowls and ornaments will polish well if vinegar is added to the washing water.

Add 15ml/1 tbsp vinegar to a small bowl of warm water. Place the item in the mixture. If the item cannot be submerged in water, then wipe it with a cloth dampened with the solution. Dry well with a clean dish towel and then polish with a clean dry cloth.

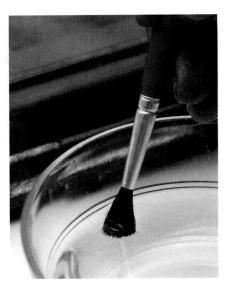

Gilt frames

To clean a gilt frame use vinegar with a very soft brush that will not scratch it.

Dust the frame, then clean with a very soft brush dampened with a mixture of 1 part vinegar to 4 parts water. Rinse the brush frequently to remove the dirt and change the water when it is dirty. Gently polish the gilt with a clean dry cloth when it is dry.

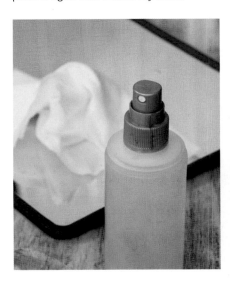

Mirrors

This is ideal for removing soapy splashes from bathroom mirrors and mirror doors.

Hold a cloth under running water, then wring out any excess water. Sprinkle a little vinegar on to the cloth and use to clean the mirror. Dry and polish with a clean cloth.

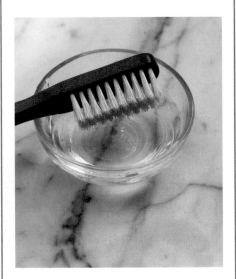

Light marble

Use a little white vinegar to remove stains from light marble.

Brush vinegar on the stained area of the marble and leave for at least 30 minutes to bleach out. Wipe the vinegar off the marble with a damp cloth.

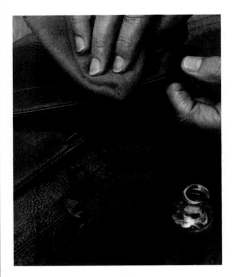

Leather

To clean, revive and preserve leather items, use vinegar and boiled linseed oil.

Mix 1 part vinegar to 3 parts linseed oil in a small bowl. Rub the mixture into the leather with a soft cloth. Polish with a clean soft duster.

VINEGAR FOR WINDOWS, WALLS AND FLOORS

Known for its ability to cut through grease, vinegar gives a bright finish to glass, mirrors and glossy paint finishes, as well as being a very effective cleaner for carpets and tiles.

Windows

This old-fashioned method for cleaning glass is well known and very effective. Using vinegar and newspaper will ensure windows are smear-free.

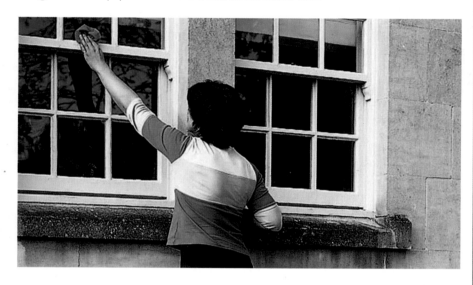

INGREDIENTS

600ml/1 pint/2½ cups vinegar

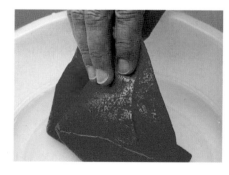

1 Soak a cloth in the vinegar.

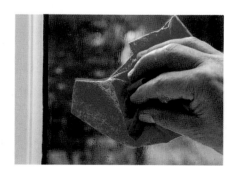

2 Clean the windows with the vinegar-soaked cloth.

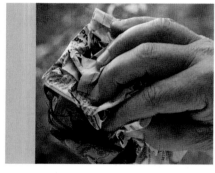

3 Rub down the windows with scrunched up sheets of newspaper.

4 If the outsides of the windows are particularly dirty, then wash well first with warm water and finish with vinegar and paper.

GREENHOUSES

This method is also excellent for greenhouses. As a simple alternative, wipe over the windows with a vinegar cloth and then polish them with a clean, dry lint-free cloth.

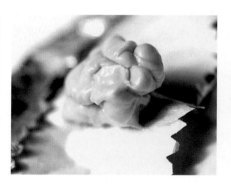

Chewing gum

Use vinegar to remove hardened chewing gum from clothing, furniture or carpets.

Test a little vinegar on a hidden area first. When applying the vinegar to fabric, soak the whole area around the gum. Warming the vinegar for a few minutes in a small pan first helps when removing gum from furniture, carpets or flooring.

Window films

These can be very difficult to remove. Take care to wipe this vinegar solution off surrounding frames to avoid damaging paintwork or varnish.

INGREDIENTS

600ml/1 pint/2½ cups vinegar

45ml/3 tbsp washing soda

1 Mix the vinegar with 600ml/1 pint/ 2½ cups boiling water in a bowl. Stir in the washing soda. Wearing rubber gloves, wash the glass with this solution. It will soften the glue so it can be rubbed off.

2 A razor blade or glass cleaning blade designed for removing paint from windows can be used to scrape off any tough bits of plastic or glue residue.

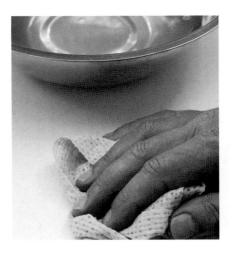

Gloss paintwork

To clean gloss paintwork, use vinegar mixed with water.

Add 250ml/8fl oz/1 cup vinegar to a large bowl of warm water and wipe the mixture over the paintwork with a damp cloth. Dry and polish the surface with a lint-free cloth. To bring a gleam to large areas of paintwork, dust and wipe down as usual, then dry with a clean cloth. Sprinkle a little vinegar on to a clean damp cloth and rub down the paintwork, then polish with a clean cloth.

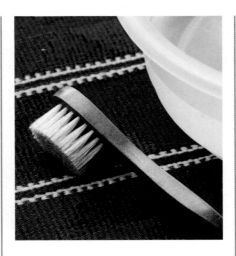

Floor rugs

Use a little vinegar in warm water to clean and restore floor rugs.

Vacuum clean, shake and/or beat the rug first to remove as much dirt and dust as possible. Brush it thoroughly. Add 250ml/8fl oz/1 cup of vinegar to a bucket of warm water. Test a little of the solution on the underneath to make sure the colours do not run. Then dampen a handbrush and brush the rug lightly all over with the solution. This will brighten colours and remove dirt.

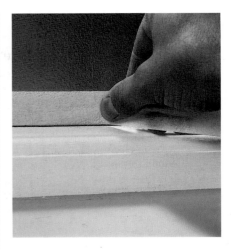

Masking tape residue

If masking tape is left on windows after decorating the frames, the glue deposit left behind can be difficult to remove.

If there is a hard, yellowed deposit that can be scraped off using a blade, do this first – use a sharp blade at an acute angle to avoid scratching the glass. Mix 600ml/1 pint/ 2½ cups vinegar and 600ml/1 pint/2½ cups boiling water in a large bowl. Stir in 45ml/ 3 tbsp washing soda. Rub on the vinegar and soda solution. Wash and repeat until all the deposit has been removed.

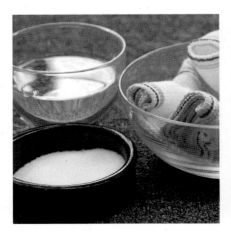

Carpet stains

Use a vinegar and salt mixture to remove light carpet stains. Test on an out-of-sight patch before use.

In a small bowl, mix 30ml/2 tbsp salt with 110ml/½ cup vinegar until the salt has all dissolved. Rub the mixture into stains, allow to dry, then vacuum.

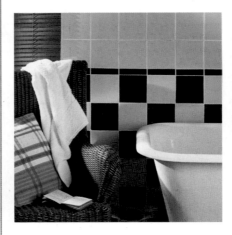

Wall tiles

Clean tiles with a damp cloth sprinkled with vinegar then polish with a dry cloth.

For thorough cleaning, for example to remove cooking splashes, rub with vinegar, then wash off with soapy water. When dry, polish with a damp cloth and a little vinegar, followed by a dry cloth.

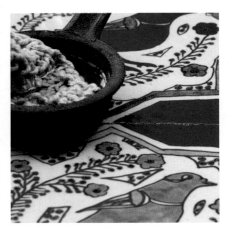

Floor tiles

Vinegar is an excellent rinse aid for the final water used after cleaning a floor.

Clean floor tiles as usual. Add 250ml/ 8fl oz/1 cup vinegar to a bucket of warm water. Use the vinegar and water mixture to give the floor a final rinse to leave it gleaming.

VINEGAR FOR FIXTURES AND FITTINGS

White distilled malt vinegar is ideal for polishing gleaming fittings but ordinary dark malt vinegar is fine for restoring older grimy metals.

Old handles

Metal furniture handles that are old and have become tarnished and filthy can be removed and cleaned thoroughly with vinegar.

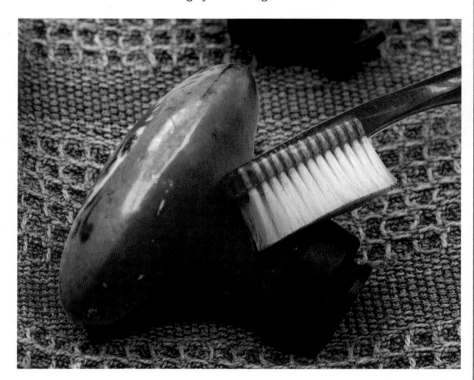

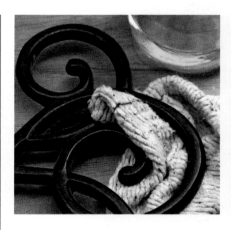

Black grates

Use vinegar to polish black fire grates or stoves.

Use a cloth dampened with vinegar for rubbing on the blacklead polish. This will remove grease and dirt and improve the quality of the polish.

INGREDIENTS

60ml/4 tbsp vinegar

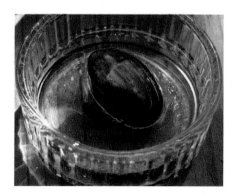

1 If the item is encrusted and very tarnished, it may need soaking briefly in vinegar. Brush off any loose dirt, then place the item in a saucer or shallow dish and pour the vinegar over it.

2 Brush the surface with a small paint brush. Remove the handle from the vinegar as soon as the metal begins to look cleaner.

Variation

Particularly dirty items can be boiled. Place in a small pan and cover with vinegar, then bring slowly to the boil. A few minutes' simmering is usually enough but the item may have to be soaked in the hot vinegar, in which case remove from the heat, cover and leave to stand. Always clean with a soft brush that will not scratch the metal, then rinse the item in hot soapy water, dry thoroughly and polish with a clean cloth.

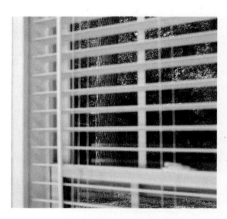

Venetian blinds

This technique works wonders on grimy Venetian or slatted blinds.

Mix together vinegar and warm water in equal parts. Briefly soak the fingers of a white cotton glove in the mixture. Put on the glove and slide your fingers along the slats of the blind, top and bottom. The dirt will come off in your hands.

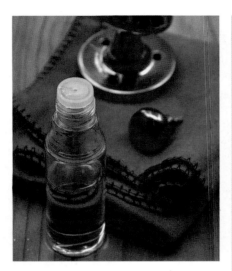

Brass fittings

This old-fashioned method was used for cleaning chandeliers or similar fine brass fittings.

Heat 60ml/4 tbsp vinegar. Fold a cloth into a pad, dip it in the vinegar and sprinkle with salt, then rub this over and around the fitting. Rinse with warm soapy water and dry thoroughly. Polish the metal with paraffin oil or a light oil, such as sweet almond oil.

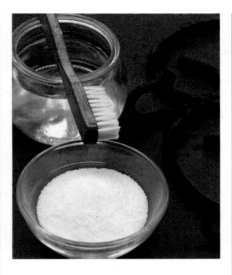

Rust

Use vinegar with salt to scrub off small patches of rust on intricate metal fittings.

Prepare two small bowls, one of vinegar, about 60ml/4 tbsp, and one of salt. Dip a stiff toothbrush in the vinegar, then in the salt and use to scrub off rust. Rinse the toothbrush in the vinegar then use to brush off the salt. Dry the metal and buff it with a clean lint-free cloth.

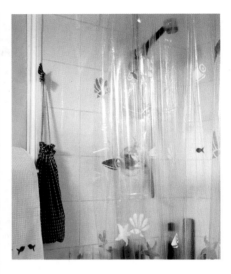

Showers

Vinegar is a great cleaner for shower heads, curtains, doors and fittings.

Clean the shower head with a solution of equal parts vinegar and water to remove deposits. Polish fittings with the same mixture and use to wipe over the tiles before buffing. Polish glass shower doors with a damp cloth sprinkled with vinegar. When washing out a shower curtain, add 50ml/ 2 fl oz/¼ cup vinegar to the final rinse.

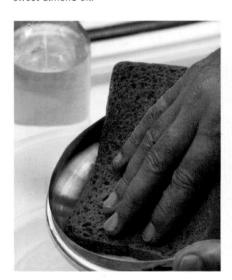

Stainless steel fittings

Polish stainless steel fittings with vinegar for a gleaming finish.

Soak a sponge in hot water and sprinkle with a little vinegar. Squeeze most of the water out of the sponge. Use the sponge to rub stainless steel handles and fittings.

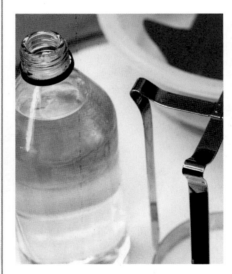

Chrome

Polish chrome items and fittings with vinegar and water.

Soak a cloth in a solution of equal parts of vinegar and water. Wring out the cloth and use to polish chrome fittings. Buff with a clean dry cloth.

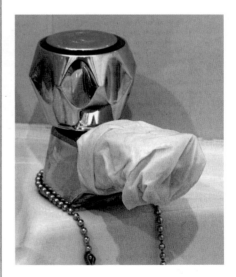

Taps

Use vinegar to remove the dirt and limescale that can build up on taps.

Soak a paper towel in vinegar for 5 minutes. Wrap around the tap. After 1 hour, remove the paper towel and clean as usual. This will remove limescale and hard water deposits.

VINEGAR FOR REMOVING ODOURS

For wiping or spraying, vinegar is a useful deodorizing agent for combating unpleasant odours around the home, from smoky fireplaces to strongly-smelling foods in the kitchen.

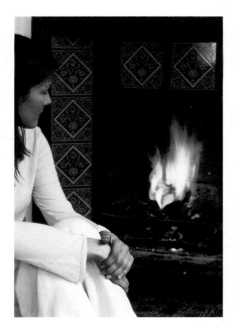

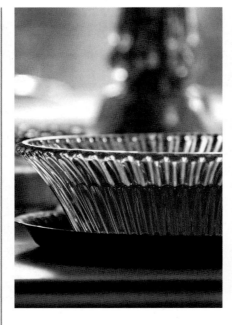

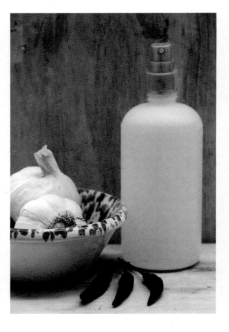

Room odours

Adding a little vinegar to hot cinders will remove the smell of smoke from a room with an open fire.

INGREDIENTS

hot (but nor glowing) cinders or charcoal
120ml/4fl oz/½ cup vinegar

1 Shovel the hot cinders into a suitable metal bucket or empty coal scuttle.

2 Place this on the hearth or other heatproof stand. Pour on the vinegar.

Variation

If the smoky smell has spread to rooms with no fireplace, heat some barbecue charcoal in a large roasting tin in the oven on the hottest setting until it is very hot. Place this on a suitable heatproof base in the room and pour over the vinegar. As the cinders or charcoal cool, any smoky smells will be neutralized.

Smoky rooms

The smell of smoke from cigarettes can often linger on soft furnishings for several days. With this simple method, all traces of the smell should be gone in less than 24 hours.

Fill a small, shallow bowl about three-quarters full of cider vinegar. Place the bowl in the room where the smell is strongest. If necessary you can use several bowls in different rooms to get rid of persistent odours.

DRAIN DISORDERS

Try using a little vinegar as a first-stage solution for dealing with slightly smelly drains. Pour 250ml/8fl oz/1 cup vinegar into the problematic drain and leave it for several hours. Flush out the drain with very hot, soapy water. Repeat the process if necessary.

Food smells

For a gentle and natural alternative to aerosol air-fresheners, try this vinegar mixture. It is particularly effective for removing strong cooking smells in the kitchen.

Mix together 5ml/1 tsp baking soda, 15ml/1 tbsp distilled white vinegar with 475ml/16fl oz/2 cups water. Transfer the mixture into a small spray bottle, and spray into rooms as required to remove odours.

GARBAGE DISPOSAL UNITS

Bits of food can get caught in the blades of garbage disposal units, causing unpleasant odours. To prevent this, make vinegar ice cubes with a mixture of one part vinegar and one part water. Run the ice cubes through the garbage disposal unit every few weeks to keep it clean and odour-free.

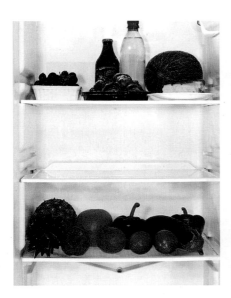

Refrigerator hygiene

The refrigerator should be cleaned regularly with a little vinegar.

Remove all the shelves and clean with hot soapy water. Give the interior a final wipe over with a damp cloth wrung out in hot water to which a little vinegar has been added. This will remove any smells and leave it fresh and clean.

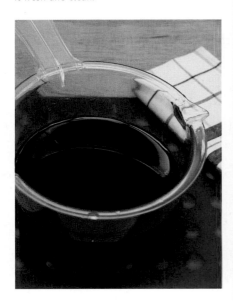

Cooking smells

Heat a small amount of vinegar on the hob to reduce food smells.

Pour a 120ml/4fl oz/½ cup vinegar into a small pan. Bring to the boil then place over a low heat, for the duration that the food giving off the smell will be cooking.

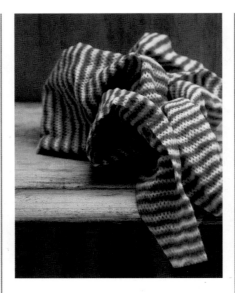

Musty cupboards

Wash cupboards and shelves out with this solution.

Add 225ml/1 cup vinegar, 225ml/1 cup ammonia and 60g/¼ cup baking soda to 4 litres/3 pints warm water. Dampen a cloth in the mixture then use to wipe down the interior of the cupboard. Leave the doors open until dry.

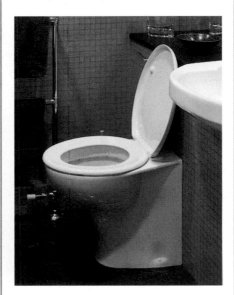

Toilets

Use vinegar to deodorize and freshen up the bathroom.

To freshen up the toilet, pour 600ml/ 1 pint/2½ cups vinegar into the bowl. Leave for at least 30 minutes before flushing the vinegar away.

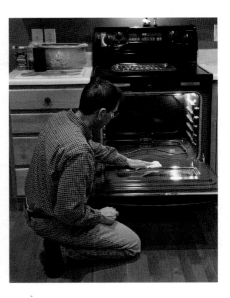

Smelly ovens

Use a mixture of equal parts vinegar and water to remove lingering odours from ovens.

Place a 120ml/4fl oz/½ cup each of vinegar and water in a suitable heatproof container in the oven and heat until it is boiling. Turn off the heat and leave the vinegar water to stand in the oven overnight. The next day, wipe the oven out with a damp cloth which has been wrung out in vinegar and water. The heated vinegar will remove odours, as well as softening any hard, dried-on food, making it easy to wipe clean.

Microwaves

Use a little vinegar to clean a microwave.

Heat equal amounts of vinegar and water in the microwave for 2 minutes, then wipe down the insides with a damp cloth.

Oven-cleaner smells

Chemical oven cleaners can have a very strong smell which may linger for several days after cleaning.

Use the oven cleaner as directed on the packaging. To neutralize any strong smells, wipe down the oven with vinegar directly after using the chemical cleaner.

VINEGAR FOR THE KITCHEN

Vinegar is an inexpensive alternative to commercial cleaning products, and can be used in a variety of ways, from cleaning cupboards to removing stains from vases and chopping boards.

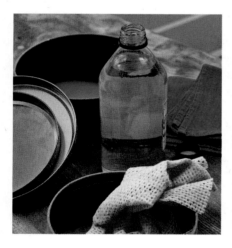

Biscuit tins and bread bins

Empty the crumbs and clean out biscuit tins and bread tins regularly.

Wipe down tins with a cloth sprinkled with neat distilled white vinegar. Leave tins open so that they dry out completely before using. This method is also good for lunch boxes.

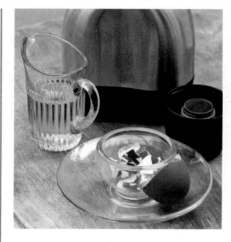

Thermos flask

Remove tainting from strong flavours.

Crush the shell of one egg and add to the flask with 15ml/1 tbsp vinegar. Cover with warm water and seal. Shake well and empty into a bowl. Repeat if necessary, then rinse well.

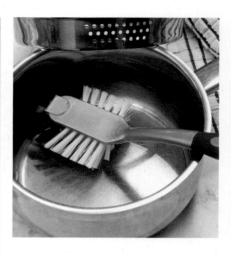

Stainless steel pans

Vinegar will leave pans gleaming.

Pour 30ml/2tbsp vinegar into a stainless steel pan and clean with a brush. Rinse with hot water. Repeat if necessary. For the outside of the pan, use vinegar on a cloth with a little salt as a scouring agent.

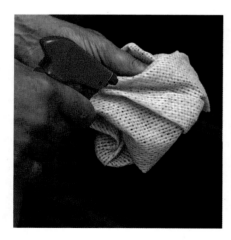

Kitchen cupboards

Wipe shelves with vinegar and water.

Fill a spray bottle with half and half distilled white vinegar and water, then use for wiping down the insides of cupboards. Leave the cupboards empty and open to dry if time allows.

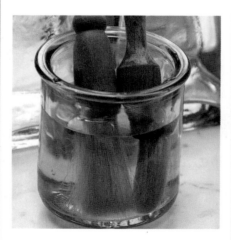

Pastry brushes

Vinegar is useful for cleaning the oil from pastry brushes.

Soak the pastry brushes overnight in a glass of vinegar. Add a little washing up liquid and work out the oil, then wash in hot, soapy water.

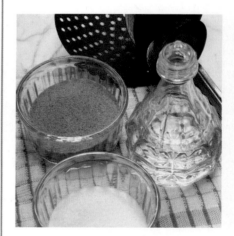

Copper pans and utensils

Bring back the sparkle to copper.

Wash the items in hot water. Use a mixture of sand and salt as a scouring agent and mix in a little vinegar to moisten. Rub over the copper with a cloth, adding more vinegar as required. Rinse with warm water.

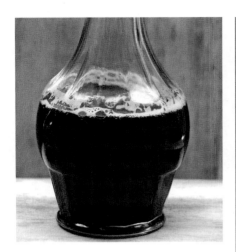

Stained vases

This is an old-fashioned cleaning method using vinegar and tea leaves. It is good for removing stains from the insides of vases.

Pour warm water into the stained vase so that it is about two-thirds full and add 15ml/1 tbsp each of vinegar and tea leaves. Shake well and leave the mixture to stand for at least three hours. Shake the mixture occasionally, checking on the progress of the stain removal. Drain the vase and rinse it out well with clean warm water.

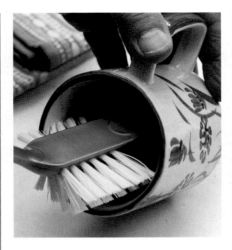

Stained mugs and cups

The insides of cups and mugs often become unpleasantly stained with tea and coffee, especially when they are not rinsed and washed immediately after use.

Pour in 15ml/1 tbsp vinegar and scrub with a washing up brush, then wash and dry. For really stubborn stains, especially on glazed pottery, scrub with a little vinegar and leave to stand for a while before rinsing. Alternatively, add a little vinegar to hot water in the mug and leave to soak for a few hours.

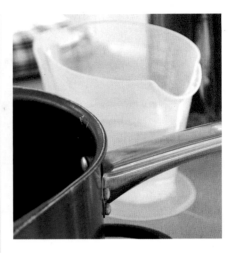

Burnt pans

Use vinegar to remove burnt-on food from the inside of pans.

If food has burnt slightly on the bottom of a pan, add 30ml/2 tbsp vinegar and a little water, to cover the bottom of the pan, then bring to the boil. Remove the pan from the heat and cover, then leave to soak to soften the burnt-on food. If the burning is fairly minor, then heating the pan with a little vinegar, allowing to cool and scrubbing is usually enough. For more severe burning, the pan may be left to soak overnight.

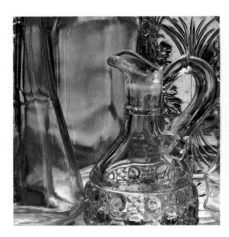

Glass carafes and decanters

This is a simple and effective approach to cleaning glass items.

Pour a little vinegar into the container, swill it around and add warm water. Leave to stand for a few hours or overnight. This is particularly useful for lightly stained items.

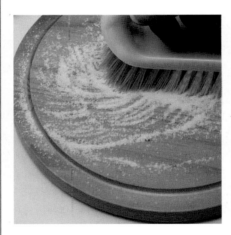

Chopping boards

Remove germs and staining from boards.

Wash boards well in hot soapy water. Drain and scrub with distilled white vinegar, sprinkling with salt for scouring, if needed. Rinse under hot water and allow to drain and dry before storing.

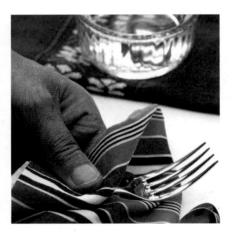

Cutlery

Clean tea or coffee stains on spoons, or water stains on stainless steel cutlery.

Dip cutlery in a little vinegar and rub with a cloth or kitchen paper. Wash in very hot water and dry immediately, polishing with a dish towel.

VINEGAR FOR LAUNDRY

Using vinegar is an old-fashioned and effective way of preventing the colour from running in bright fabrics. It has several other laundry uses too.

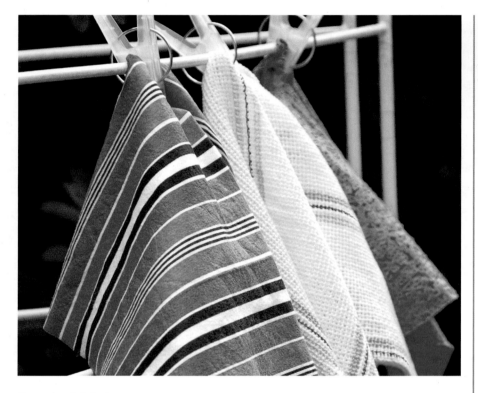

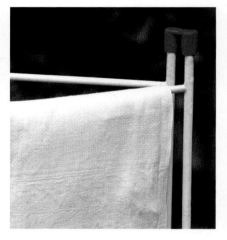

White fabric
Use vinegar to whiten yellowed fabric.

Wash and rinse the fabric. Rinse out in a little vinegar and water, and hang out in bright sunlight to dry.

Scorched fabric
This will remove scorch marks caused by ironing cotton or linen. Fuller's earth clay is available from craft shops.

INGREDIENTS

30ml/2 tbsp soap trimmings or soap flakes
2 large onions, peeled and grated
20ml/4 tbsp fuller's earth clay
250ml/8fl oz/1 cup vinegar

1 Place the soap trimmings or soap flakes in a pan and add 250ml/8fl oz/ 1 cup of water.

2 Heat gently, stirring, until the soap has completely dissolved.

3 Place the grated onions in a sieve (strainer) over the pan. Press out the juice from the onion into the dissolved soap.

4 Add the fuller's earth clay and the vinegar to the soap and onion mixture and stir well. Bring to the boil, then remove from the heat, stir well and cover. Leave to cool.

5 Spread out the scorched area of fabric, laying it over a pad of cloth or on a plastic rack. Spread the cooled mixture over the scorch mark and leave it to dry completely. Then wash out the fabric and let it dry in bright sunlight.

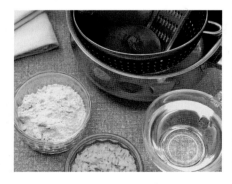

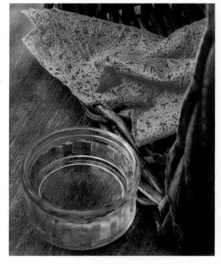

Laundry baskets
This is particularly useful for cleaning basketwork items.

Wipe down the inside of laundry baskets with a damp cloth sprinkled with a little vinegar. Leave to dry completely before using.

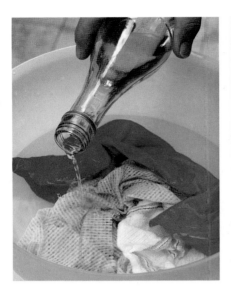

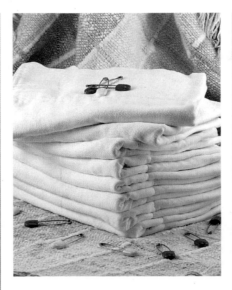

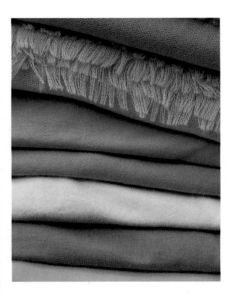

Dishcloths, brushes and sponges

If a dishcloth is to be left unused for some time, or after clearing up at the end of the day, use vinegar for a thorough clean.

Rinse out cloths in a bowl of water with a little vinegar added. Open out and hang up to dry. Rinse brushes and sponges in water with vinegar added, shake off or wring out and leave to dry.

Terry nappies (diapers)

Place dirty terry nappies in a bucket of water and vinegar to soak before washing. This will neutralize odours.

Add 300ml/½ pint/1¼ cups distilled white vinegar to a 5-litre/1-gallon bucket water, and leave the nappies to soak until it is time for them to be washed. When it is time for the nappies to be washed, drain the vinegar water, rinse and wash as usual.

Coloured fabric

Just as vinegar restores colour to red cabbage that has been steeped in salt before pickling, vinegar can also be used to brighten up washed-out fabric.

Wash clothing as usual. Add 250ml/8 fl oz/ 1 cup vinegar to rinsing water to restore colour. The acid in the vinegar is mild enough so that it will not harm clothing, but strong enough to dissolve alkalines in detergents.

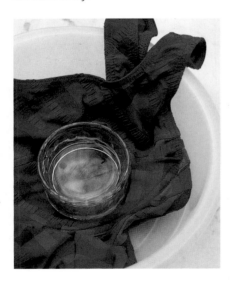

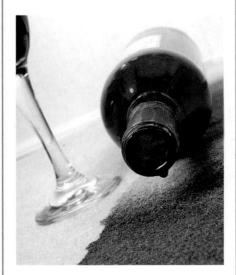

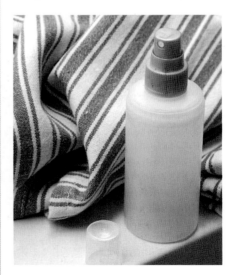

Swimwear

Use vinegar to clean swimwear and remove the chlorine smell that comes from swimming in public pools.

Wash out swimwear in soapy water. Rinse in water with a little vinegar added – this will remove any traces of chlorine.

Wine stains

This works best if done within 24 hours of staining.

Sponge neat white distilled vinegar on to the affected areas and rub away the stains. Wash according to the garment's care instructions.

Fabric shine

After ironing, dark fabrics can develop a shine. White vinegar will remove this.

Transfer a little vinegar to a spray bottle. Spray a little on to the affected area, then sponge off with cold water. Test a small hidden area of fabric first.

VINEGAR FOR DECORATING

Grease-free surfaces are vital for good results when decorating and vinegar is the ideal cleansing agent during the preparation stages.

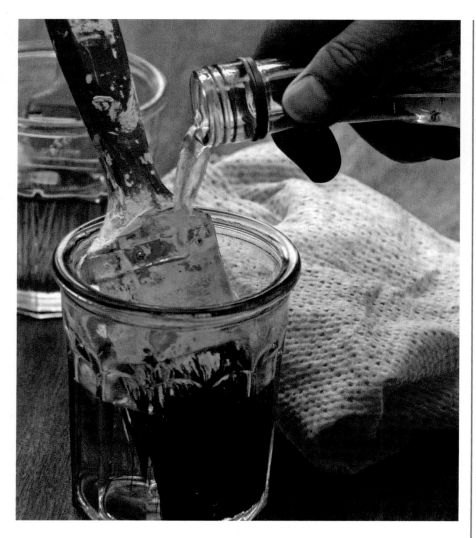

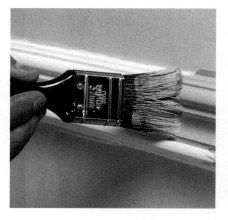

Woodwork preparation

When freshening up woodwork with a coat of paint, use vinegar to clean off grease and dirt first.

Pour a little vinegar on to a cloth and wipe down all woodwork which is to be painted. Then wipe with water, using a damp cloth, and dry thoroughly with paper towels. Sand down the surface ready for the new paint.

Wallpaper

If washing soda is used to strip wallpaper, use a vinegar solution to neutralize it so that it does not soak in and discolour new layers of paintwork.

To neutralize the soda solution, wipe down the walls with a vinegar solution, one part vinegar to two parts water. Leave to dry completely before sanding down and continuing with the painting.

Paint brushes

Depending on the type of paint and severity of the build-up, vinegar can be an effective relatively mild cleaner.

INGREDIENTS

250ml/8fl oz/1 cup vinegar

washing soda

1 Soak the paint brushes up to the tops of their bristles in the vinegar for several hours or overnight, then wash out with detergent and hot soapy water.

2 If the paint build-up is severe, the best way of cleaning brushes is by soaking them in a strong solution of washing soda overnight. This will release dried paint and soften the top of the bristle area.

3 Wear rubber gloves and use detergent to lather out all the paint into the soda solution. Rinse the brush in hot water.

4 Finish by soaking in a vinegar and water solution to neutralize any remaining soda. Rinse thoroughly, shake out and leave to dry.

DECORATING ODOURS

Place small dishes of vinegar around a room while decorating, to reduce the potency of odours from paint or varnish.

VINEGAR FOR PET CARE

Always check out traditional home cures for pet problems with your vet when in doubt – many encourage simple vinegar home remedies.

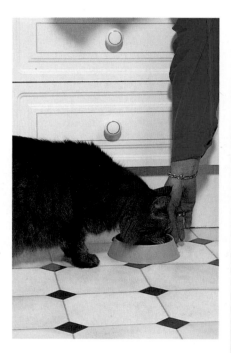

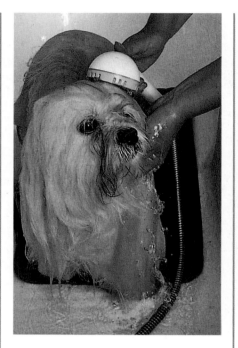

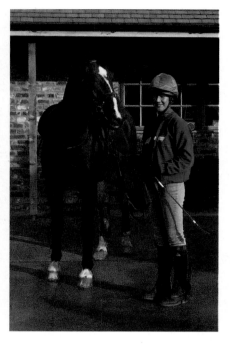

General pet tonic

Cider vinegar is recommended as a tonic for pets, given in small doses in the drinking water. The idea is to introduce the cider vinegar gradually so that the animal becomes accustomed to the slightly acidic flavour of the drinking water. It is said to be beneficial to cats, dogs and rabbits as well as horses. Including cider vinegar in the diet deters ticks and fleas.

Many vets encourage an organic approach to pet care and will be happy to offer advice on how to supplement a particular pet's diet in this way.

1 Start by adding 1.5ml/¼tsp cider vinegar to the pet's drinking water.

2 Gradually increase the amount of vinegar until you are adding 5ml/1tsp.

Cider vinegar pet wash

Washing pets with cider vinegar is said to help prevent flea attacks. Check with your vet for expert advice on exactly the right proportion to use.

Add a few drops of vinegar to the pet's regular bath water. Make sure that you rinse it off well afterward with warm water.

Pet litter trays

Even after a thorough cleaning, plastic pet litter trays can sometimes retain unpleasant odours.

Rinse the pet litter tray out with white vinegar, scrub well with a brush and rinse again with the vinegar. Be sure to rinse the tray out well afterward in clean cold water – a fussy pet will refuse to use litter that still smells of vinegar. Leave to dry in the open air.

Horse grooming and care

Adding a little cider vinegar to foodstuff and/or grooming a horse with garlic vinegar is an effective way of keeping flies off. Vinegar can be used to clean the horse's legs after removing mud or to treat sweet itch, and can also help prevent the horse from scratching any irritating bites.

Pet hutches and cages

Rabbit hutches and the cages of other small pets, such as hamsters or mice, can be cleaned out with distilled white vinegar.

Clean the animal's hutch or cage as usual. Wipe out the inside of the hutch with white vinegar. This will neutralize any odours. Wipe the hutch down again, this time with clean water, to remove any lingering smell of vinegar. Allow to dry before replacing any bedding.

VINEGAR FOR THE CAR AND GARDEN

Cut down on costly, environmentally unfriendly chemicals by using vinegar outside your home, in the garden and to clean your car.

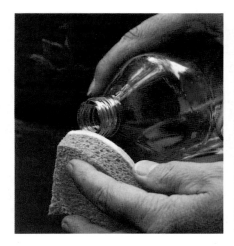

Flowerpots

Use vinegar to clean and remove build-ups of mould from flowerpots that have been left outside.

Scrub unglazed flowerpots with a little neat vinegar to remove any mould or growth. Wash thoroughly and allow to dry.

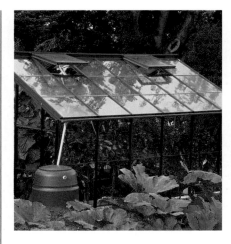

Greenhouse

Use vinegar to clean greenhouse glass.

Use a soft brush to brush vinegar on to the glass, then scrub with crumpled up newspaper. Wash down with water and rinse with a bucket of water to which 250ml/8fl oz/1 cup of vinegar is added.

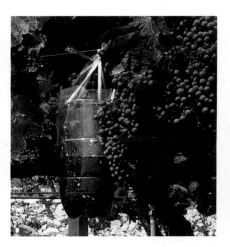

Insect trap

A mixture of vinegar and apple juice will attract insects and keep them off plants.

Put 250ml/8fl oz/1 cup each of vinegar and apple juice in a container. Hang near plants you want to protect. Insects will be lured to the vinegar mixture and away from plants.

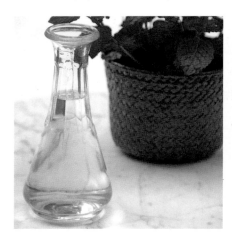

Insect deterrent

Use vinegar as an insect deterrent on potted plants where adding acid to the soil is not a problem.

Add a few drops of vinegar to the soil, taking care not to get any on the plant itself. Water the plant as usual.

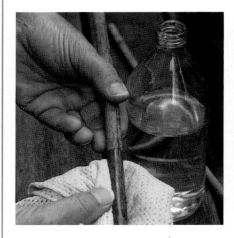

Poles and plant supports

Prevent garden canes, poles and plant supports going mouldy while they are in storage.

Wipe down with neat vinegar when removing poles from plants. Leave to dry completely before storing.

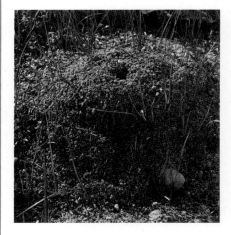

Ant deterrent

Once you have rid a nest of ants, deter them from returning with vinegar.

Pour boiling water on an ants' nest and all around the surrounding area. Once dry, pour vinegar around the area to stop the ants returning.

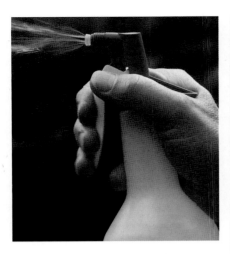

Garden sprayers

Vinegar can be used to clean out weedkiller from the insides of a garden sprayer.

Add 250ml/8fl oz/1 cup each of water and vinegar to an empty garden sprayer after rinsing out the weedkiller. Shake thoroughly and spray the mixture through the nozzle to clear it. Leave to stand overnight, then rinse thoroughly. If in any doubt, read the instructions for the particular weedkiller used in the sprayer to check that it will be neutralized by the acid in the vinegar.

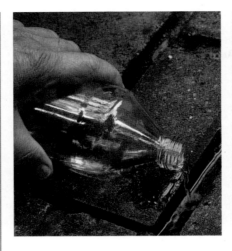

Weed deterrent

Use vinegar to clean paving slabs and as a weed deterrent around pathways and doorsteps.

Remove all weeds and brush the slabs down to remove all loose dirt. Add 475ml/16fl oz/2 cups vinegar to a bucket of warm water and use to scrub down paving slabs. If the slabs are especially stained, green or dirty, spray neat vinegar all over them and leave to soak before scrubbing down. Drizzle neat vinegar around the slabs and steps to prevent the weeds coming back.

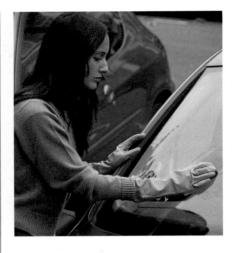

Car windscreens

Use vinegar and toothpaste for a crystal-clear windscreen.

Wash the car windscreen down with warm water, then use a little toothpaste as a mild abrasive to clean the glass, then rinse off with water. Add 120ml/4fl oz/ ½ cup vinegar to a bucket of warm water, wring out a cloth and wipe the windscreen with the vinegar and water mixture. Polish with a chamois leather before it dries. Take care not to get vinegar on the car's paintwork as it may damage it.

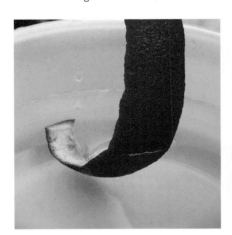

Cat repellent

To overcome a cat-spraying problem, use a combination of orange peel and vinegar.

Dip strips of orange peel in vinegar and place them around the cat's favourite spraying place. Keep spraying the peel with vinegar until the cat has moved on to a new place.

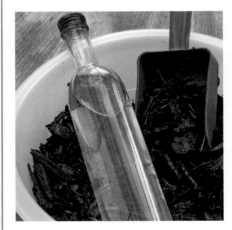

Slug barrier

A barrier of vinegar-soaked chippings around plants will deter slugs.

Soak wood chippings in vinegar and place around beds of seedlings. Maintain with vinegar top-ups. Do not flood the area – it will kill the plants.

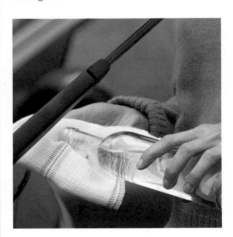

Windscreen wipers

Remove the greasy build up on windscreen wiper blades with vinegar.

Pour a little white vinegar on to a cloth. Clean the windscreen wipers with vinegar. This will remove grease and also stop them from squeaking.

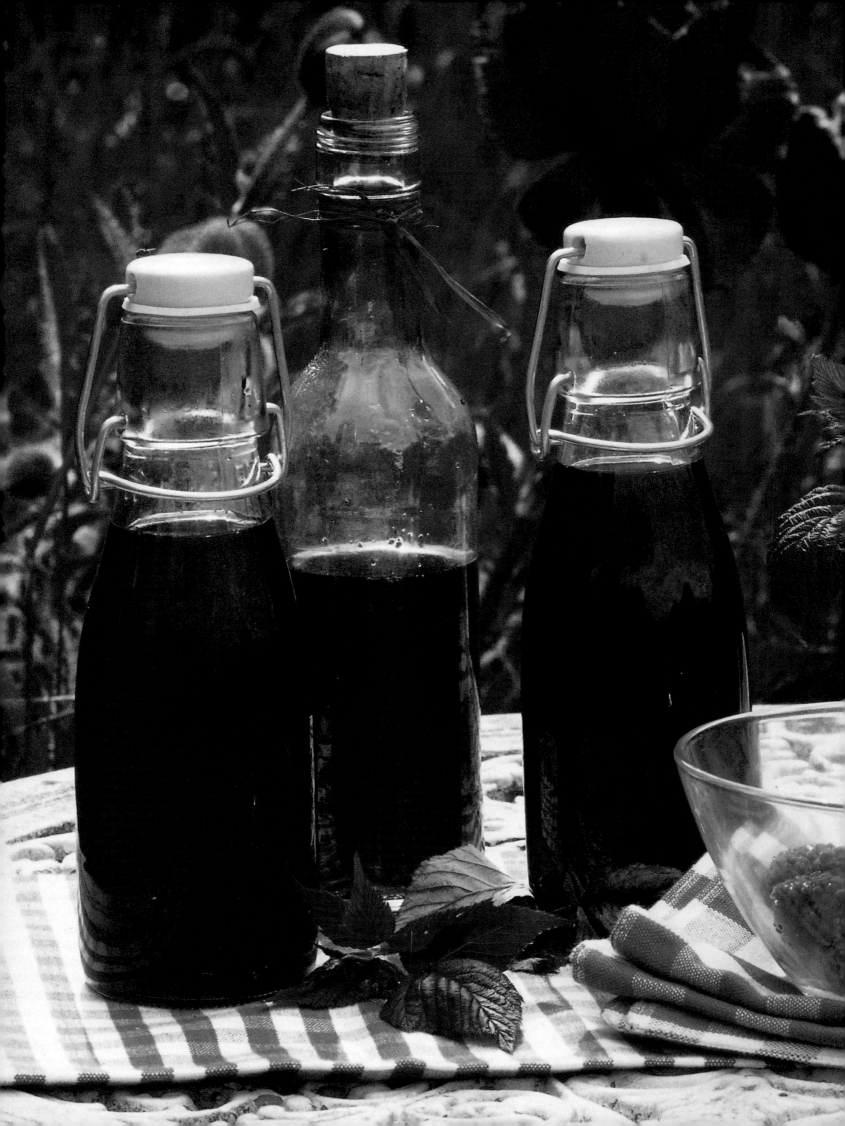

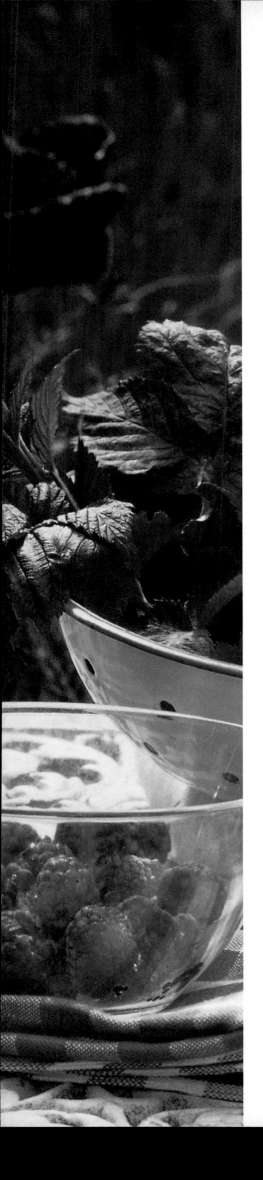

VINEGAR IN THE KITCHEN

Various types of vinegar are used for all sorts of cooking. While many methods are steeped in history, others are comparative newcomers to the culinary scene. Whether it is used for marinating, dressing, deglazing, sharpening, flavouring, or even raising cakes, the addition of vinegar will enrich and improve many dishes. From essential food preservation techniques to frivolous finishing touches, vinegars of one sort or another should feature in every cook's repertoire.

Left: Preserve the essence of fresh fruits and herbs by making your own flavoured vinegars.

CULINARY USES OF VINEGAR

Versatile vinegar plays several essential roles in classic cuisines from around the world, from food cleaning and preparation, to flavouring, marinating and of course preserving.

Basic types of vinegar can be used throughout the processes of preparing, cooking, preserving and serving food. The array of fine-flavoured, and often expensive, vinegars now widely available are usually used to add the finishing touches to dishes, to flavour drinks or, quite simply, served as dipping sauces.

Vinegar in food preparation

Removing strong flavours Vinegar is used to rinse or soak food that naturally has an odour or for removing, or reducing, strong flavours that have developed when food has deteriorated slightly (but not to the extent of being inedible). For example, fresh skate has a slight smell of ammonia and washing in water acidulated with vinegar removes or reduces this. Rinsing with vinegar also counteracts slightly rancid flavours, for example if fat that is tainted is removed from poultry or meat, the meat can be rinsed in vinegar to remove any residual flavour. Venison fat (of which there is not usually very much) has a bad flavour and rinsing in vinegar after trimming off any fat and membrane removes any residual flavour. Vinegar is also used in the preparation of tripe to clean it and remove unpleasant flavours.

Cleaning Vinegar is used in the first stages of food preparation to clean produce. Adding a little vinegar to a bowl of water in which fresh garden lettuce and other leaves

are washed brings out insects and bugs that otherwise manage to conceal themselves throughout several rinses. The method also works well for wild berries, such as blackberries, that tend to harbour tiny maggots.

Vinegar is often used with salt to prepare snails. The freshly gathered snails are purged (fed on herbs or starved) for about a week in a box with a finely perforated lid to rid them of any remnants of poisonous plants. They are washed and then sprinkled with salt and vinegar. This process is repeated until the snails are free from slime, when they are boiled and shelled ready for using.

Preventing discolouration Placing peeled fruit and vegetables that tend to discolour in cold water with a little vinegar added prevents the items from

changing colour while the rest of the batch is prepared. For example, this is useful when preparing potatoes, artichokes, apples and pears.

Marinating and macerating Vinegar can be used to marinate savoury ingredients or macerate fruit. The choice of vinegar depends on the type of dish and whether it will be used in a sauce or discarded. The majority of marinades and soaking mixtures are either used in the cooking liquid, to baste food or served in a sauce.

When macerating fruit, the vinegar usually acts as a dressing or sauce, or it is used in a syrup. Fine wine vinegars or fermented fruit vinegars are ideal for macerating fruit to be served raw and the acidity of the vinegar brings out the flavour of fruit, such as strawberries or papaya, that do not have a high acid content.

Above: Adding vinegar to water when washing salad will remove insects.

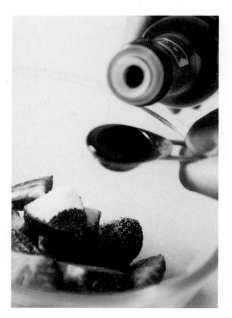

Above: The acidity in balsamic vinegar enhances the flavour of certain fruits.

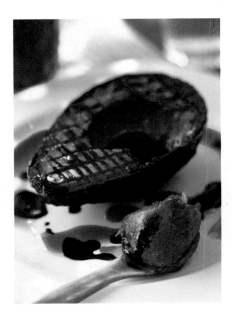

Above: Vinegar is commonly used with oil as a dressing or finishing ingredient.

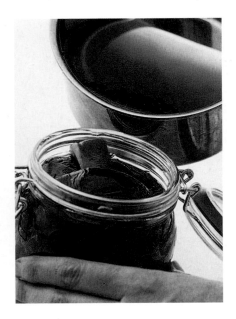

Above: Vinegar has been valued for its preservation properties for centuries.

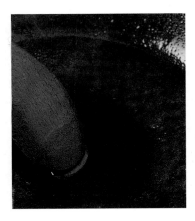

DEGLAZING WITH VINEGAR

Cider or wine vinegars are often used to deglaze cooking pans, either after frying, grilling (broiling) or roasting.

Balsamic vinegar is probably one of the most popular vinegars for this process, but all sorts of vinegars are useful, including fruit vinegars, spiced and herb vinegars. The important thing is that the harshness of the vinegar balances the food or other ingredients that may be added to a sauce. Rich, mellow, sweet-sour vinegars can be used to deglaze the pan and complete the dish without the need for any other ingredients. On the other hand, deglazing with a sherry vinegar, brown rice vinegar or cider vinegar can bring just the right level of piquancy to a gravy or rich wine sauce.

When you are deglazing a pan, add comparatively small quantities of liquid in one go and keep scraping, whisking or stirring the sediment and juices off the pan.

Control the heat to avoid burning the sediment or the vinegar. This is particularly important when using rich and sweet vinegars, such as balsamic.

Sauces made by deglazing are often left concentrated in flavour and modest in volume, so a little is drizzled over each portion. Instead of coating food with a larger quantity of lighter sauce, this allows for pleasing contrasts when eating the main dish and vegetables or salad, for example, as flavours and textures come through individually.

Vinegar in cooking

Balancing strong flavours A little vinegar is often added to the poaching liquid for strongly flavoured fish and is also used in court bouillon, a cooking liquid used for fish.

Sharpening One of the main contributions vinegar makes to food is to add a sharp flavour. When food is bland or without any hint of acidity, a little vinegar accentuates the flavour and brings out the characteristics of the ingredients, typically with fruit, such as blueberries, but also with vegetables, such as beetroot (beets). Flour-based sauces may be slightly sharpened with a hint of vinegar or it can be used to bring contrast to soups and gravies.

Cutting richness Vinegar is excellent for balancing the richness of dishes and foods that have a high fat content. Examples include egg-based sauces and in roasting juices or sauces for rich and fatty main foods, such as duck or lamb.

Setting eggs Adding vinegar to water when poaching eggs helps to set the whites quickly.

Raising agent The chemical reaction between vinegar and baking soda serves as a raising agent in some traditional baking recipes.

Vinegar in preservation

The preservation properties of vinegar are fundamental to its culinary value and it is for this purpose that vinegar is used in the largest proportion. It is used in a wide variety of preserves, with ingredients ranging from fish to fruit, and from simple pickles that require minimum preparation to more sophisticated jellies and store sauces.

Vinegar in finishing and dressing

Added to a cooking pan after frying or roasting food, vinegar is used to loosen the residue and incorporate the juices and some fat in a sauce or gravy (this is called deglazing). However, the simplest use of vinegar is as a straightforward dressing or condiment. It is drizzled over cooked or raw food or dishes to add piquancy and contrast. Partnered with oil it is used for a variety of dressings.

VINEGAR IN DRESSINGS AND MARINADES

When used in dressings, vinegar adds a tangy kick to vegetables and salads. Meat, fish or poultry are tenderized by vinegar marinades, ready for cooking.

On its own or partnered with oils and herbs, vinegar is the classic dressing ingredient. There is nothing easier than drizzling rich balsamic vinegar over a green salad. Simple oil and vinegar salad dressings need little introduction – they are as familiar and popular as mayonnaise. Home-made vinegar dressings are easy to mix and keep well in the refrigerator.

Beyond the salad

Vinegars and dressings do not have to be reserved for salads – they are also terrific on grilled (broiled), pan-fried, stir-fried, steamed or poached foods. Use favourite vinegar dressings instead of rich milk or cream sauces or high-fat gravies to bring pleasing piquancy and contrast to fish, poultry or meat. Drizzle a little dressing over boiled new potatoes or cauliflower instead of butter or cheese sauce. Top with a few Parmesan shavings for a hint of cheese. Toss freshly boiled or steamed green or runner beans with a little dressing instead of loading them with butter.

Marinating with vinegar

Vinegar is used in marinades to tenderize meat. The vinegar may be used with water or wine and the proportion is usually relatively small. This type of marinade is popular for all meats and game (especially venison). The flavouring ingredients (spices, herbs, onion, carrot) are usually heated with a little water, wine or vinegar first so that they release their flavour, then allowed to cool. More marinating liquid may be added. When cooled, the food to be marinated is added and turned in, or basted with, the mixture.

Marinating time depends on the type of food, dish and intensity of flavour required – it can be anything from 30 minutes to 3 days. For short

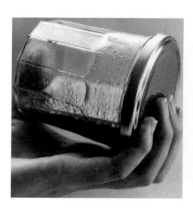

VINEGAR DRESSING TIPS

When you are making a vinegar-based dressing, always start with the vinegar, dissolving all the flavourings and seasonings in the vinegar. Salt, sugar or mustard, for example, should be mixed into the vinegar first until dissolved. A good way to do this is to place all the ingredients together in a screw-top jar and then shake them up. Then the oil should be added. This way the seasonings sing through the whole dressing rather than separating out as sediment at the bottom.

Pick the vinegar and oil to suit the main ingredients in the dish, and to suit personal preferences – mild cider vinegar makes a super-soothing dressing compared to a more piquant wine vinegar.

Using vinegars flavoured with fruit or herbs can completely change the appearance of a salad, turning a simple plate of green leaves into a dish of flavour contrasts, for example.

For a well-balanced oil and vinegar mixture, you should use one part vinegar to two parts oil.

Not all dressings need oil. Try a simple dressing of rich balsamic vinegar or sweet raspberry vinegar, with a little citrus zest and some ground black pepper.

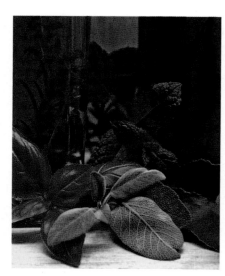

Above: Herb vinegars give extra flavour to salad dressings and marinades.

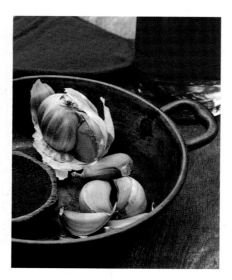

Above: Vinegars flavoured with garlic or spices make great salad dressings.

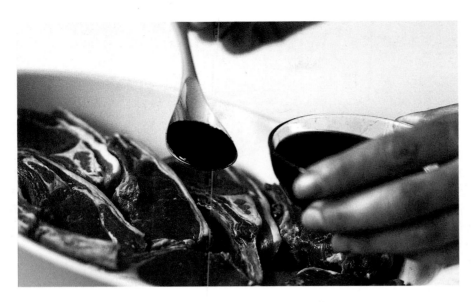

Above: Marinating lamb chops in rich balsamic vinegar for several hours before they are cooked will leave the meat tender and moist.

BASTING

Marinades should always be heated if they are used for basting. This avoids cross contamination from the raw, unheated mixture in which the raw meat has been marinating to the finished cooked food. It is particularly important when brushing a marinade over grilled (broiled) food, such as chicken or turkey.

If the marinade is not brought to the boil after marinating, bacteria from the raw food may be brushed over the grilled food just before serving.

marinating the food is left covered in a cool place but not chilled; for longer marinating the food is placed in the refrigerator. When left for any length of time, the food should be turned occasionally or regularly to ensure that it is evenly flavoured.

The food may be drained before cooking, for example when grilling (broiling), roasting or barbecuing. The marinade may be used for basting or glazing during or after cooking, or it may be included in the cooking liquid, for example when making a casserole, braising or pot roasting. Alternatively, it may be added to, or heated as, a sauce at the end of cooking.

Matching vinegar with ingredients

Key points to consider are the strength of flavour of the food and any other ingredients, whether it is served raw or cooked and the required finished flavour, particularly in terms of tartness or sweet-sour balance.

Fitting the vinegar to the food means selecting according to how sharp it is, whether it has a clear 'brisk' sharpness without any supporting fruitiness, richness or sweetness.

While some flavour characteristics survive in hot dishes others are completely lost. The distinct sherry characteristics of some sherry vinegars are good in hot sauces and balsamic vinegar will clearly flavour roasted vegetables, but the flavour of blueberry vinegar or an aromatic moscatel vinegar is diminished drastically when used in cooking.

In macerating or marinating the pronounced flavours of some vinegars permeate and are balanced by main ingredients, but the delicate fruitiness of other vinegars is diluted. Fermented fruit vinegars (as opposed to fruit-flavoured vinegars) are perfect for drizzling over just before serving when their flavours will still be fresh and clear, without marinating or macerating, and no cooking.

When vinegars are drizzled over immediately before serving and not stirred in, even though they may be fruity or relatively delicate in flavour, they may well match foods or dishes that are quite heavily spiced or flavoured with herbs. Instead of being incorporated, they bring occasional contrast as the food is eaten.

MARINADE INGREDIENTS

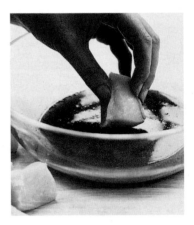

Cider or wine vinegars are used for marinades: light ones for fish and poultry, red or darker ones for meat and game.

Fruit vinegars make excellent marinades, adding flavour interest. Some unpasteurized fruit vinegars (such as pineapple vinegar) have strong tenderizing properties if they retain the enzyme from the fruit that gradually breaks down protein.

Typical spices that are used for marinating red meat include juniper berries (good with game), coriander, cloves, mace (the blade of mace rather then the ground spice) and cinnamon sticks.

The most suitable herbs for marinating include rosemary, thyme, oregano and sage. Dill and fennel are often used in lighter marinades, with white wine or cider vinegar.

VINEGAR AND PRESERVATION

One of the key culinary uses of vinegar has always been, and still is, as a preservative, especially for fruit and vegetables in pickles and chutneys.

One of the first uses of vinegar was as a food preservative. Being able to preserve food during times of plenty for periods of scarcity was essential for survival. Right up until modern technology provided practical, affordable alternatives by way of refrigerators and – especially – freezers, every cook relied on vinegar for preserving summer produce for winter meals. Preserves may no longer provide an essential source of sustenance for winter but they are an inherent part of the cuisines of all countries. They bring intense, contrasting flavours to simple meals, they enliven burgers, grills and barbecues and add a burst of flavour to sandwiches and filled breads.

How it works

Cooking foods with, or immersing them in, vinegar creates an acidic environment that is not suitable for the growth of the majority of micro-organisms that cause food spoilage. This is the easiest method of making preserves and it is used particularly for vegetables and fruit. The sharpness of the vinegar is often balanced by adding sugar, creating a sweet-sour flavour, and the high proportion of sugar in many preserves also helps to prevent spoilage.

Mature flavours

The majority of vinegar preserves should be allowed to mature before they are eaten. This allows time for the spices, herbs and other flavourings to penetrate

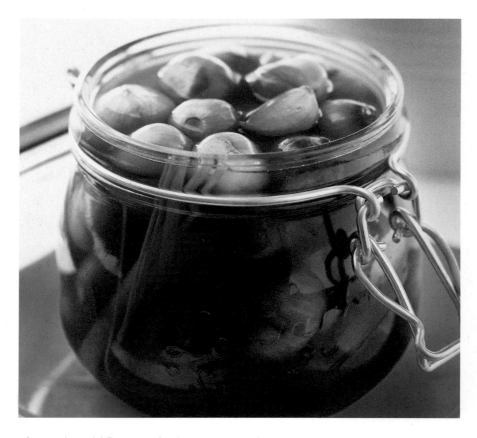

Above: The mild flavours of cider vinegar or white wine vinegar work well when pickling strong-tasting ingredients such as these aromatic Thai pink shallots.

the main ingredients. Individual flavours mingle and mellow, linked by the sharp or sweet pickle. Rich strong preserves that are intended to keep for up to 2–3 years taste better after 1–3 months' maturing, whereas others that taste best eaten within 6 months are usually ready after 2–3 weeks' maturing.

Keeping qualities

Ingredients which have been preserved in vinegar keep very well for long periods, with deterioration in texture or colour being the usual limiting factors rather than drying out or micro-organism attack. As long as

all the equipment used is thoroughly cleaned, the ingredients properly prepared and measured, and the cooking method followed, foods preserved in vinegar will keep for years. The jars or bottles have to be properly covered and stored in a cool dark place.

Before the food becomes mouldy or develops off flavours, it is likely to soften in texture (or, in the case of eggs become very rubbery) and look discoloured. The natural flavour of the ingredients may also diminish in intensity, so even though the food is safe to eat it will not taste its best.

Types of vinegar preserves

As a preservative, vinegar is used in savoury recipes, including pickles, chutneys, sauces, ketchups, relishes and jellies. Sugar is often used to counterbalance the sharp taste, giving a sweet-sour flavour.

Pickle This may be simple pickled ingredients, such as vegetables, preserved in plain or spiced vinegar. The basic ingredients may be raw or cooked. Additional flavouring ingredients can be added or the vinegar can be sweetened. When choosing vinegar for sweet pickles, it is important to think about the colour as well as the flavour of the vinegar. For green fruits such as green figs or red fruits such as plums, choose a light-coloured vinegar and spices or flavourings that won't alter the colour. Using a dark vinegar will turn the fruits a sludgy brown colour. Yellow fruits such as nectarines and apricots, and white or creamy fruits such as pears, look stunning pickled in a coloured vinegar such as raspberry. As well as vegetables, fish, eggs, fruit and unripe walnuts can be preserved by pickling.

Pickle is also the term used for a mixture of ingredients, usually cut into chunky pieces, and preserved in a vinegar-based sauce. The ingredients are usually cooked, either in the pickle liquid or before they are immersed in the sauce. Piccalilli is a classic example – it consists of mixed vegetables cooked in a sweet-sour mustard and turmeric sauce – but any chunky equivalent of a chutney could be called a pickle.

Chutney Chutney is the term for a cooked preserve. Onions, garlic, spices and other flavouring ingredients are combined with fruit and/or vegetables, then cooked in vinegar until thick and rich. Sugar is added to balance the flavour. As a rule, a chutney has a finer texture than a pickle and it is cooked for longer. Some chutneys are long cooked and well reduced.

Relish Relish refers to the sweet-sour and/or spicy flavour of the preserve, which is usually finer in texture than a pickle but not as smooth and thick as a chutney. Chilli and/or other hot spices may be used in relishes but some are mild, for example corn relish is sweet-sour and mild.

WHICH VINEGAR TO USE?

The acidity of the vinegar is essential for effective preservation and it should contain 4–6 per cent acetic acid. The flavour is important and diluted acetic acid condiments posing as vinegar are not suitable for preserving (or for any other culinary purpose as their flavour is poor).

Malt vinegar is a favourite for its acidity and flavour; it is also less expensive than wine or cider vinegars and therefore more practical for use in large quantities. Brown malt vinegar is good in rich chutneys and pickles, but its colour is unacceptable for some preserves. Light malt or white vinegars may be used when a lighter colour is important. Malt vinegar can be purchased ready spiced for pickling but the flavour is very mild.

Cider vinegar is a good choice for cooked pickles, chutneys and relishes where a milder flavour is required. Similarly, when more modest quantities of vinegar are used in a recipe, wine vinegars can bring excellent flavour to relishes and chutneys, or to pickled fruit.

Jellies These are essentially fruit and sugar preserves, similar to jams and sweet jellies. Vinegar is used to make sweet-sour herb or fruit jellies to complement meat or cheese. Apple, lemon and mint jellies are typical.

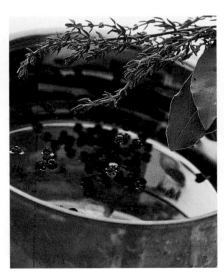

Above: Brown malt vinegar is the best choice for use in rich chutneys.

Above: White vinegar can be bought ready-spiced or spiced at home for pickling.

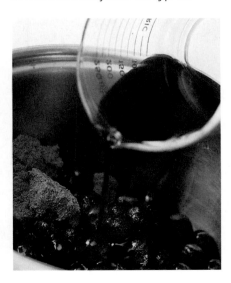

Above: When pickling fruit, think about the colour as well as the taste of the vinegar.

CULINARY TRICKS WITH VINEGAR

Vinegar is useful in the kitchen for improving the performance of ingredients or enhancing simple mixtures in a wide variety of ways.

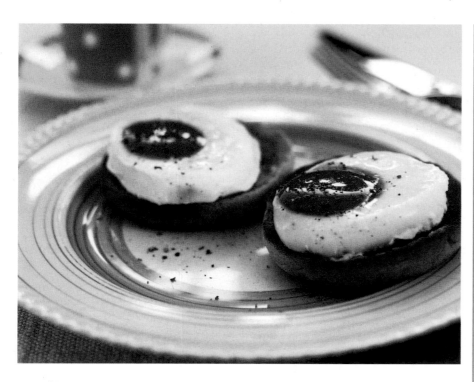

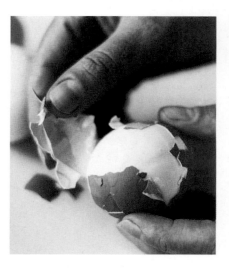

Peeling eggs

Adding a little vinegar to water makes it easier to peel hard-boiled eggs when they are cooked.

Add 5ml/1 tsp vinegar and 15ml/1 tbsp salt to boiling water before gently placing the eggs into the water.

Poaching eggs

Adding vinegar to the poaching water makes the whites set more quickly.

INGREDIENTS

5ml/1 tsp vinegar

1 egg

English breakfast muffins, to serve

2 Poach the egg for 2–3 minutes in the barely simmering water. This will leave the yolk soft and runny. The circular swirl of water keeps the egg white in good shape, preventing it from spreading in strands, and the vinegar helps to set it quickly.

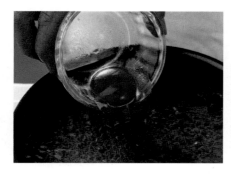

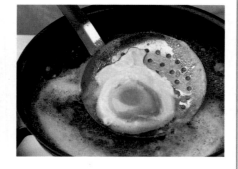

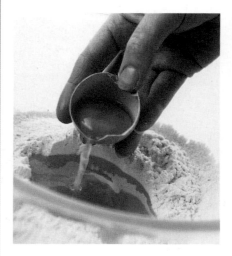

1 Add 5ml/1 tsp vinegar to a pan of water and bring to the boil. Reduce to a simmer. Crack an egg into a cup, swirl the water with a spoon, then slip the egg into the middle of the swirl.

3 Carefully remove the egg from the water using a slotted spoon.

4 Serve immediately with buttered English breakfast muffins.

Making eggs go further

This is an old-fashioned suggestion for making one egg do the work of two.

When baking a cake, use 15ml/1 tbsp vinegar with 1 egg instead of adding 2 eggs.

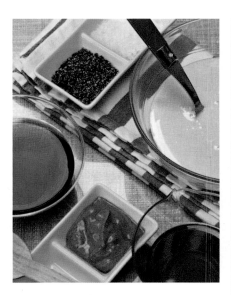

Making salad cream
From a 1930s cookbook by Elizabeth Craig, this was suggested as a good alternative to mayonnaise.

Pour a small can of evaporated milk into a large bowl and alternately mix in 250ml/ 8fl oz/1 cup vinegar and 30ml/2 tbsp vegetable oil. Add a little salt, pepper and mustard to taste.

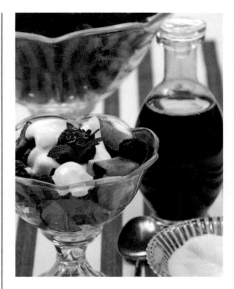

Using vinegar in sweet dishes
Use sweetened fruit vinegars and balsamic vinegar to dress fruit for dessert. Serve alone or with cream or yogurt.

Drizzle balsamic vinegar over pan-fried or grilled (broiled) fruit, such as bananas, peaches or pears. Serve fruit vinegars with plain vanilla mousse, cheesecake or ice cream for a tangy contrast.

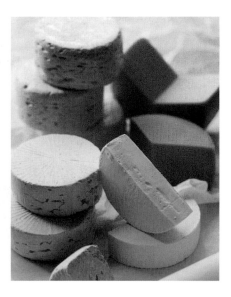

Storing cheese
Wrapping cheese in a vinegar-soaked cloth before storing it in the refrigerator will keep it fresh and moist.

Place a little vinegar in a bowl. Soak a clean cloth or paper towel in the vinegar. Squeeze out most of the liquid, then use to wrap the cheese. Place in an airtight container and store in the refrigerator.

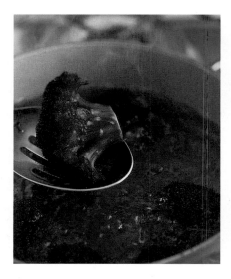

Preserving colour of vegetables
Adding a little vinegar to the water will improve the colour of boiled vegetables.

Bring a large pan of water to the boil, then add 15ml/1tbsp vinegar before carefully placing the vegetables in the water and cooking as usual. This will help them to retain their colour.

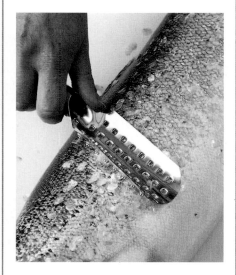

Descaling fish
Rubbing fish skin with vinegar will make it easier to remove the scales.

Place a little vinegar in a small bowl and rub it into the fish skin with your fingers. Leave for 5 minutes, then descale the fish as usual. The vinegar will also help to reduce any fishy odour.

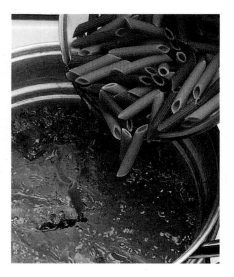

Cooking pasta
Adding vinegar to the cooking water will prevent pasta from being sticky.

Bring a large pan of water to the boil. Instead of adding salt, add 5ml/1tsp vinegar. Add the pasta and cook as usual. The addition of the vinegar will reduce the starch and make the pasta less sticky and easier to serve.

FLAVOURING VINEGARS

A wide variety of commercially produced flavoured vinegars are available, but it is easy and fun to try making your own. Use vegetables, herbs, spices and even flowers.

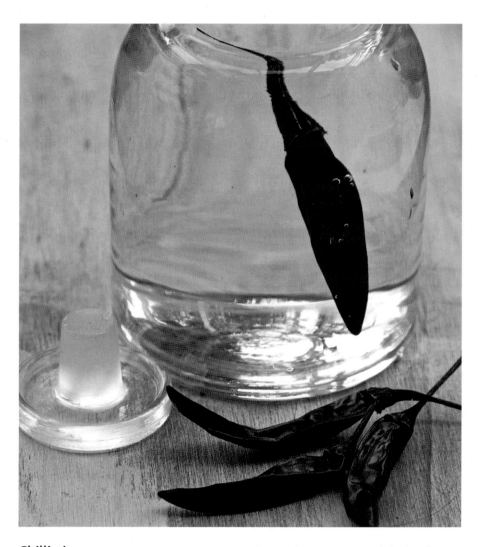

FLAVOURING VINEGARS AT HOME

There are endless possibilities for flavouring vinegars at home, from spicing inexpensive vinegar for pickling to flower-scented vinegars and vibrant fruit vinegars. Flavouring vinegar is not that difficult to do at home and it is a good way of preserving the essence of fresh garden herbs or local seasonal fruit.

Experiment with fresh garden produce, lively herbs and favourite spices to make a range of vinegars that can be used to infuse exciting flavours into salad dressings and sauces.

The choice of vinegar depends on its likely uses. Malt may be ideal for pickles and chutneys but not practical for salad dressings, sauces or marinades. Wine vinegar will go well in some dressings or for deglazing a cooking pan but may be too harsh for dressing a fruit dessert.

Cider vinegar will be useful for dressings, sauces and drinks. The recipes here are a mixture of traditional and modern, and intended to spark off ideas for experimenting with flavouring and using a variety of different vinegars.

Chilli vinegar

Easy to make with dried or fresh chillies, this chilli vinegar can be added to many dishes to give them that extra bite. It makes a great addition to pickles, chutneys and sauces, and will add a touch of fiery colour when drizzled on to salads, pasta dishes and pizzas.

INGREDIENTS

1–2 dried red chillies, or 1–3 fresh green or
  red chillies, halved and deseeded
1 bottle of vinegar

1 Pour the vinegar out of the bottle and reserve. Place the dried or fresh chillies in the bottle then refill with the vinegar. Seal.

2 Leave the chilli vinegar to infuse in a cool, dark place for anything from a week to 6 months.

Variation

Deseed and finely dice 1 red (bell) pepper and add it to the vinegar with the chillies to make a fiery pepper chilli vinegar.

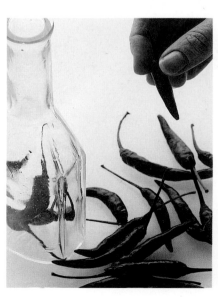

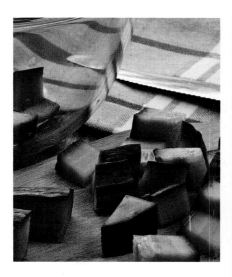

Cucumber vinegar

The fresh taste of cucumber makes this a perfect vinegar to use in salad dressings.

Dice a cucumber and layer it in a bowl with a light sprinkling of salt. Leave for at least 3 hours to draw out the excess water. Drain and squeeze out the cucumber, then place in a clean dry bowl. Pour in enough vinegar to cover generously. Cover and leave to stand for 3 days before straining and bottling.

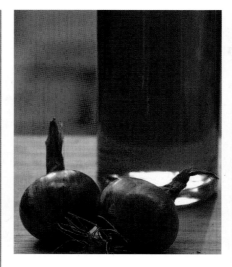

Shallot vinegar

A traditional accompaniment to oysters, this is best made with wine vinegar.

Add a finely diced shallot to a bottle of vinegar. Seal and infuse (steep) for 1–2 weeks, then strain and bottle. Alternatively, flavour bottles of vinegar with trimmed and chopped spring onions (scallions) or chives. Chinese garlic chives can also be used to make a strongly flavoured vinegar.

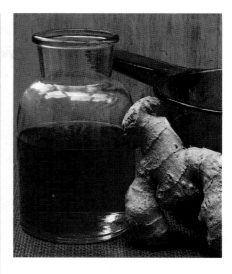

Ginger vinegar

Use this in oriental cooking, in stir-fried dishes or dipping sauces.

Finely chop a piece of fresh root ginger, about 4cm/1½in. Simmer the ginger in 5cm/2in vinegar in a covered pan for 30 minutes. Cool before transferring to a glass container, then pour on enough vinegar to fill. Seal and infuse for about a month, then strain and add sugar to taste before bottling.

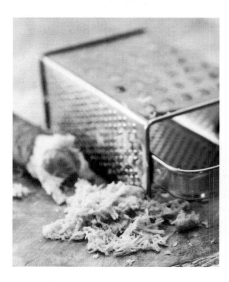

Horseradish vinegar

Add a little horseradish vinegar to gravy and serve with roast beef.

Scrub and grate 115g/4oz fresh horseradish. (Horseradish is very strong so wear gloves.) Put the grated horseradish in a glass bottle and cover with vinegar. Seal and infuse (steep) for at least a week before straining and bottling.

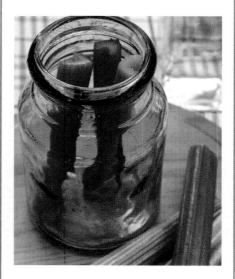

Celery vinegar

This can be added to soups, sauces or salad dressings.

Slice 1–2 celery stalks lengthways. Place the celery in a jar, without packing in tightly. Pour in vinegar to cover, shaking out all the air, cover and leave to stand for 3–4 weeks. Strain and bottle the vinegar.

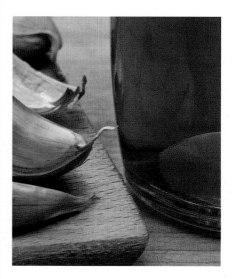

Garlic vinegar

Use this to make delicious marinades for fish, shellfish and chicken.

Peel and halve one large or two small cloves of garlic, then add the garlic to a bottle of vinegar. Seal, and leave to stand for at least a week, then strain and bottle the vinegar.

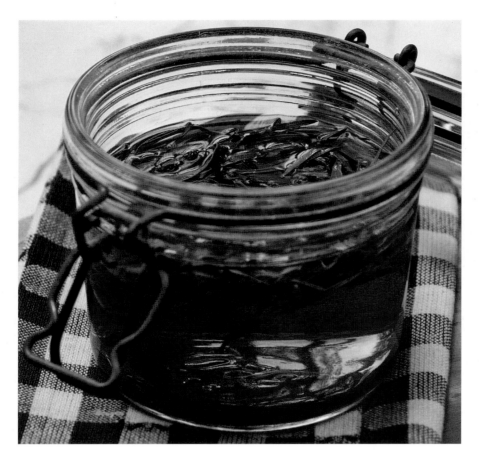

Herb vinegars

A wide variety of herbs can be used to flavour vinegar, either individually or mixed. Tarragon is the traditional choice – tarragon vinegar is a classic ingredient for salad dressings and egg sauces.

INGREDIENTS

about 15g/1/2oz/3/4 cup fresh tarragon
450ml/3/4 pint/scant 2 cups vinegar

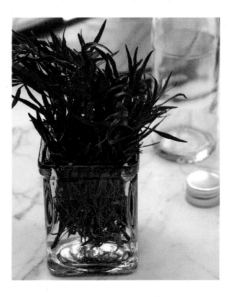

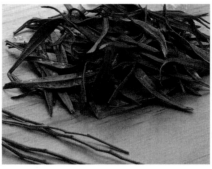

1 Wash and dry the tarragon and remove the leaves from the stalks.

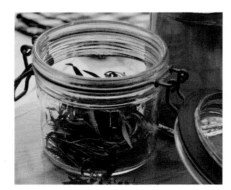

2 Place in a container and pour on the vinegar. Seal and leave to stand for 4 weeks in a cool, dark place. Strain, bottle and cover.

HERB VINEGARS

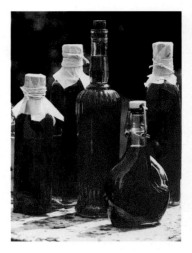

• Mint, basil, bay leaves, dill, thyme, marjoram and rosemary all impart a full flavour to wine or cider vinegars for use in sauces and dressings as well as for pickling.

• Cider vinegar is best for making herb vinegar. White or red wine vinegars are also acceptable, but malt vinegar, including light or white, is too harsh and strongly flavoured for herbal use.

• Herbs used for making flavoured vinegars should be picked in the morning after the dew has dried, but before the flavours have dissipated in the hot sun. Allow the moisture to dry completely before use, otherwise they may become mouldy.

• Herb vinegars should be strained, but you can add a few fresh sprigs of herb when bottling to indicate the flavour.

• Attractive bottles of herb vinegars make excellent gifts. Look out for interesting bottles to decant your vinegar into and use ribbons and labels for decoration.

• Try the following combinations to flavour white or red wine vinegar or cider vinegar:
    Sage, thyme, bay and marjoram
    Sage, thyme and basil
    Sage, dill and coriander (cilantro)
    Basil, thyme and oregano
    Lemon grass and rosemary
    Coriander, chives, dried
      chillies and garlic

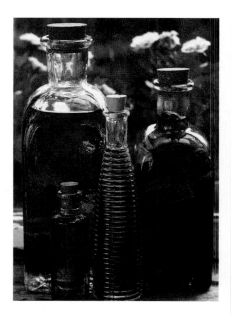

Rose petal vinegar

For a really decadent dressing, make this with Champagne vinegar.

Pull the rose petals from 2 or 3 scented rose heads. Snip off the bitter white heel at the base of each petal. Place 2 handfuls of petals in a large glass jar or bottle. Fill the jar or bottle with Champagne or white wine vinegar, seal very tightly with a screw-top or cork and leave on a sunny window sill for at least 3 weeks before straining.

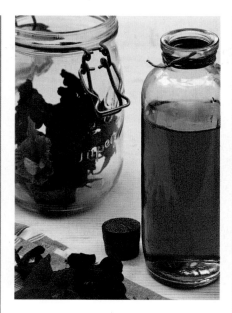

Nasturtium flower vinegar

Serve this as a dressing for salads containing nasturtium flowers.

Place a handful of nasturtium flowers in a jar, filling it without squashing the flowers. Pour in wine vinegar to cover, gently agitate the jar to remove trapped air and cover. Leave to mature for 2 months. Strain the vinegar through muslin (cheesecloth), squeezing out all the vinegar from the flowers.

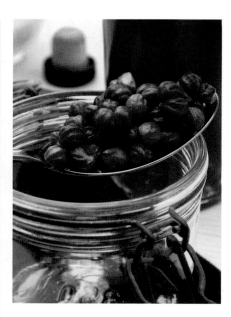

Pickled nasturtium seeds

The seeds can be used as a flavouring ingredient in a similar way to capers.

Layer 75g/3oz nasturtium seeds in a large bowl and sprinkle with salt. Leave for 24 hours, then rinse and drain well. Dry the seeds well on a dish towel and place them in clean jars without packing them in too tightly. Pour in vinegar to cover. Seal and allow the seeds to mature for at least 2 months before using both the vinegar and the seeds.

MAKING FLOWER VINEGARS

You should always be certain that flowers are edible before putting them to food use in vinegars as some flowers can be poisonous. Common edible flowers include nasturtium, rose, pansy, citrus blossom, lilac, violet and honeysuckle.

Whenever using flowers for flavouring or cooking, it is best to pick them in dry weather and early in the day, when the flowers have opened but have not had time to wilt in the sunshine. Select perfect examples and shake off any insects. Try to avoid washing the flowers as this can bruise and damage them.

Make these flower vinegars with mild flavoured vinegars – use white wine vinegar or cider vinegar for the best results.

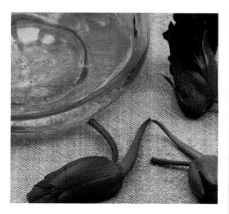

Pickled nasturtium buds

These buds have a peppery taste that is great in salads.

Pick 15–20 buds in dry weather and lay them on a paper towel for 3 days in a cool dry place. Place in jars and cover with boiling vinegar. Allow to mature for 3 months before using. Both buds and vinegar can be used.

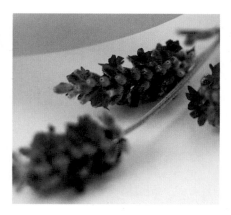

Lavender vinegar

This is delicious when used in dressings or drizzled over roast meats.

Trim the ends off several stalks of lavender and add to a bottle of vinegar. Shake to dislodge air bubbles, cover and leave to stand for 6 weeks. Strain through muslin (cheesecloth) and store in clean bottles.

Raspberry vinegar

One of the favourites, this is simple to make with fresh or frozen raspberries. There is little point in buying raspberry flavoured vinegar when it can be made so easily at home using a favourite wine or cider vinegar and just the right hint of sweetness.

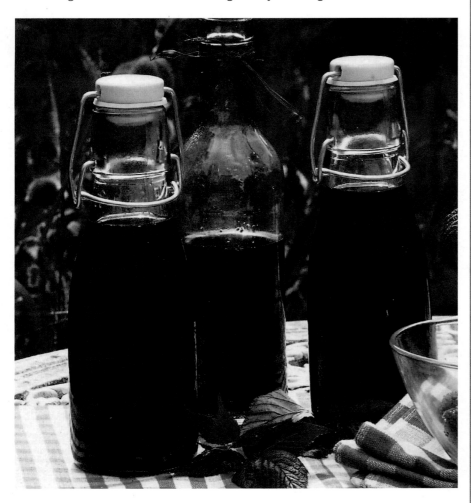

INGREDIENTS

450g/1lb raspberries, fresh or frozen

1.2 litres/2 pints/5 cups vinegar

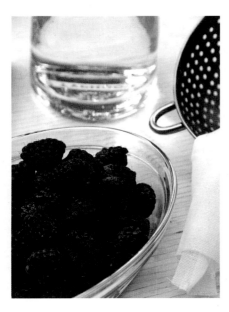

1 Macerate the raspberries in the vinegar for about 5 days.

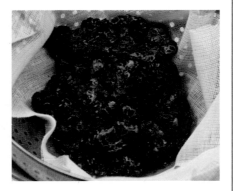

2 Strain through a sieve (strainer) lined with muslin (cheesecloth).

3 Heat with 450g/1lb sugar until dissolved, then bring to the boil. Bottle, cover immediately and cool.

FRUIT-FLAVOURED VINEGARS

These can be made in modest amounts using fresh, frozen or canned fruit. Leave unsweetened or add sugar to taste. When there is a glut of fresh fruit to use, then large quantities can be prepared, allowing about 2.25kg/5lb fruit to 2 litres/3½ pints vinegar.

White vinegar can be used for preparing large quantities but cider and wine vinegars can give better flavours and are practical for making smaller quantities. The fruit should be left to stand in the vinegar for 5–7 days before straining. When making small quantities to be used relatively quickly, there is no need to heat the vinegar. When preparing a large volume for long-term storage, the vinegar should be boiled before storing otherwise it will ferment with time.

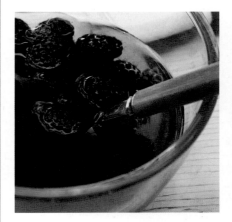

Brandied raspberry vinegar

The following old-fashioned recipe makes a rich raspberry vinegar.

Measure the raspberries by volume and add twice the volume of vinegar to the raspberries. Leave to stand for a day, then strain. Add the same quantity of raspberries and leave to stand for a further day. Strain again into a large pan and add 450g/1lb sugar to every 600ml/1 pint/2½ cups raspberry vinegar. Bring to the boil, stirring until the sugar has dissolved, reduce the heat and simmer for 1 hour. Skim off any scum as the vinegar simmers. Measure the reduced vinegar and add about 250ml/8fl oz/1 cup brandy to every 600ml/1 pint/2½ cups vinegar.

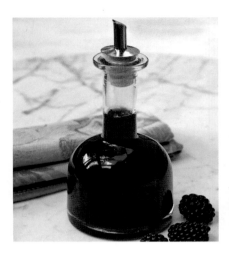

Rich blackberry vinegar

Mixed with sparkling water and a sprig of mint, this makes a refreshing drink.

Measure a jug (pitcher) of blackberries and add the same volume of vinegar. Cover and stand for 1 day. Strain, add another jug of berries, cover and leave for a further day. Strain and repeat again. Strain and add 450g/1lb sugar for every 600ml/1 pint/2½ cups vinegar. Heat until dissolved, then bring to the boil. Reduce the heat and simmer for 30 minutes. Bottle and allow to mature for 4 weeks before using.

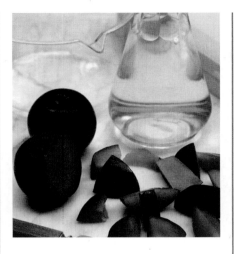

Stone (pit)-fruit vinegar

This can be made with any stone-fruit, such as sloes, damsons or plums.

Use 100g/3¾oz. To break down the skins and flesh slightly, place the fruit in the freezer overnight. Pit the fruit and chop the flesh then place in a pan, pour on 600ml/1 pint/2½ cups vinegar and bring to the boil. Cool and leave to stand for 1 week, crushing the fruit with a vegetable masher. Strain and add a little sugar to sweeten if required before bottling.

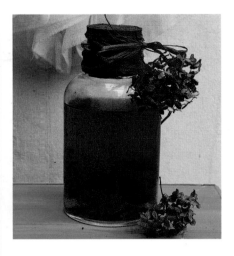

Citrus vinegar

This tangy vinegar makes a great marinade ingredient for fish dishes.

Pare off the thin outer rind of an orange, lemon or lime using a vegetable peeler. All the white pith should be removed as it will taste bitter. Place a few strips of the peel in a bottle of vinegar and allow to infuse for 3–6 weeks. Using a mixture of different coloured fruits will give an attractive result. Alternatively, add the grated zest of 1 lemon, lime or orange to a bottle of vinegar.

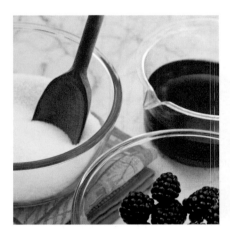

Simple blackberry vinegar

Use this method if you don't want to wait for the vinegar to infuse.

Place 100g/3¾oz fresh blackberries in a bowl, add 600ml/1 pint/2¾ cups vinegar, then leave for 2 days. Strain and transfer to a pan. Add 450g/1lb sugar to the vinegar, heat until dissolved, then bring to the boil. Simmer until the vinegar is reduced by half. Bottle.

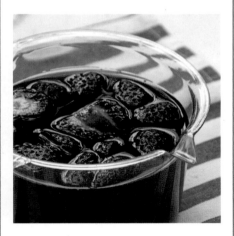

Strawberry vinegar

This has a rich and fruity flavour and is great drizzled over ice cream.

Follow the same method as for brandied raspberry vinegar (see previous page), substituting strawberries for the raspberries and without adding the brandy at the end. Adding several batches of fruit gives the vinegar an excellent rich flavour.

EASY FRUIT VINEGARS

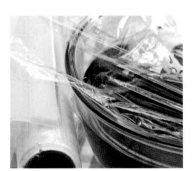

Prepare the fruit, discarding inedible parts, and cut into small pieces. Try peaches, nectarines, apricots, cherries or mango. Place in a glass mixing bowl and pour in vinegar to cover. Cover with cling film (plastic wrap) and macerate in the refrigerator for up to a week, stirring daily. Strain and sweeten the vinegar. Instead of discarding the fruit, cook down to a chutney or pickle with onions, spices, vinegar and sugar.

VINEGAR IN DRESSINGS

Vinegar is an essential ingredient in all sorts of dressings, whether you wish to add an edge to creamy dressings or a sharpness to classic combinations of herbs and oils.

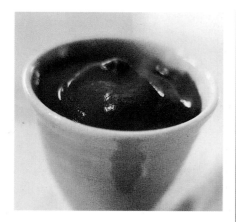

Classic vinaigrette

Make sure all the ingredients are at room temperature to make a smooth emulsion.

Put 30ml/2 tbsp balsamic vinegar in a bowl with 10ml/2 tsp Dijon mustard, salt and ground black pepper. Whisk to combine. Slowly drizzle in 90ml/6 tbsp olive oil, whisking until the vinaigrette is smooth and blended.

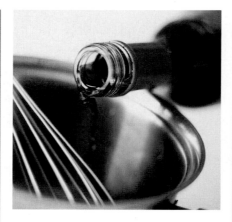

Garlic raspberry dressing

Adding a splash of raspberry vinegar to this dressing enlivens a simple salad.

Fry 2 finely sliced garlic cloves in 45ml/ 3 tbsp olive oil until just golden. Remove with a slotted spoon and drain on kitchen paper. Pour the oil into a bowl and whisk in the raspberry vinegar. Season with salt and ground black pepper.

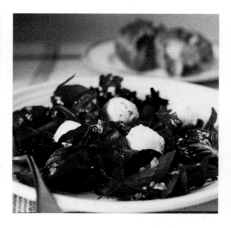

Hazelnut dressing

Serve this simple dressing with a goat's cheese salad and chopped hazelnuts.

Put 30ml/2 tbsp hazelnut oil in a small bowl. Add 5–10ml/1–2 tsp sherry vinegar or good wine vinegar to taste, and whisk the oil and vinegar together thoroughly. Season to taste with salt and ground black pepper.

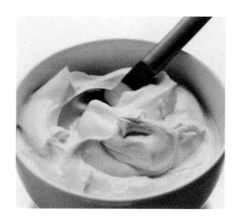

Creamy raspberry dressing

Raspberry vinegar gives this quick dressing a refreshing, tangy fruit flavour.

Mix 30ml/2tbsp raspberry vinegar with 2.5ml/ 1/2tsp salt and stir until dissolved. Stir in 5ml/ 1 tsp Dijon-style mustard and 60ml/4 tbsp natural (plain) yogurt.

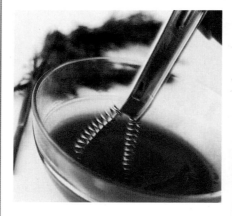

Dill dressing

Serve this simple mixture of oil, vinegar and dill with smoked fish.

Whisk 90ml/6 tbsp olive oil and 30ml/ 2 tbsp white wine vinegar together, or shake in a screw-top jar. Blend in 15ml/ 1 tbsp chopped fresh dill and season.

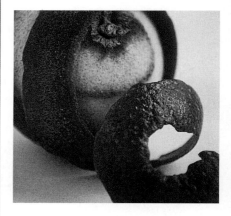

Creamy orange dressing

This tangy orange dressing is delicious with a mixed green salad.

Pour 45ml/3 tbsp crème fraîche and 15ml/ 1 tbsp white wine vinegar into a screw-top jar with the grated rind and juice of 1 orange. Shake until combined, then season to taste.

VINEGAR IN MARINADES

Using vinegar in marinades helps to tenderize meat and fish and bring out the flavours of other ingredients. Use a simple herb-flavoured vinegar or try these recipes.

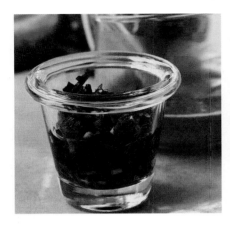

Summer herb marinade

Raid the herb garden to make this fresh-tasting marinade.

Mix 45ml/3 tbsp tarragon vinegar, 1 crushed garlic clove and 2 finely chopped spring onions (scallions). Whisk in 90ml/ 6 tbsp olive oil, then add a large handful of chopped fresh herbs such as thyme or parsley and mix well. Season.

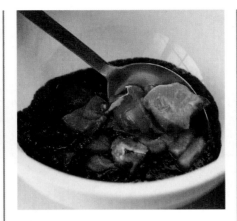

Hoisin marinade

Use this Chinese marinade for chops and chicken pieces.

In a small bowl, combine 175ml/6fl oz/ 1 cup hoisin sauce, 30ml/2 tbsp each sesame oil, dry sherry and rice vinegar, 4 chopped garlic cloves, 2.5ml/½ tsp soft light brown sugar and 1.5ml/¼ tsp five-spice powder.

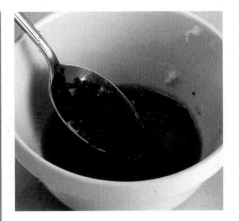

Red chilli marinade

Spice up meat and fish with this hot and fiery marinade.

Mix 2 chopped, deseeded fresh red chillies with 1 clove crushed garlic, 1 tsp ground black pepper, 60ml/2fl oz white wine vinegar, 15ml/1 tbsp caster (superfine) sugar, 30ml/2 tbsp sunflower oil and 15ml/1 tbsp freshly chopped parsley.

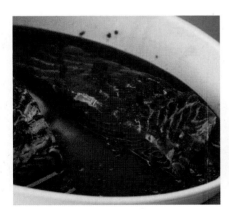

Teriyaki marinade

In this traditional Japanese recipe, soy sauce is paired with rice vinegar.

In a small bowl, combine 1 crushed garlic clove, 5ml/1 tsp grated fresh root ginger, 30ml/2 tbsp dark soy sauce and 15ml/ 1 tbsp rice vinegar.

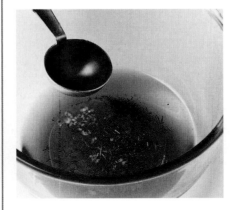

Thyme marinade

The cider vinegar in this herby marinade brings out the full flavour of the thyme.

Combine 90ml/6 tbsp olive oil with 30ml/ 2 tbsp cider vinegar, 1 crushed garlic clove, 5ml/1 tsp dried thyme and 2.5ml/½ tsp crushed peppercorns.

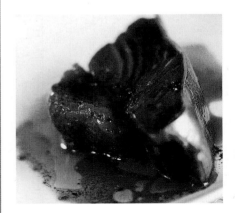

Sherry vinegar marinade

This piquant mix of sherry vinegar and garlic oil would suit fish or meat.

Mix together 30ml/2 tbsp sherry vinegar with 45ml/3 tbsp garlic-infused oil and season with salt and ground black pepper to taste.

VINEGAR IN SAUCES

Vinegar serves a sharpening and/or mixing function to add piquancy or bring flavours together effectively in many classic sauces.

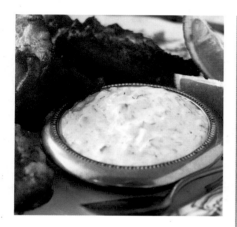

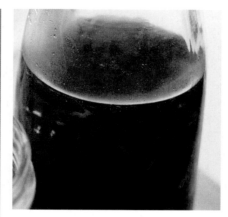

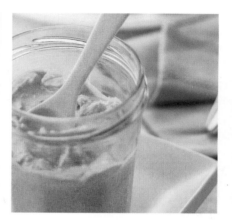

Tartare sauce

This creamy sauce is the traditional accompaniment to fish dishes.

INGREDIENTS

Makes about 475ml/16fl oz/2 cups

1 egg yolk

15ml/1 tbsp white wine vinegar

30ml/2 tbsp Dijon-style mustard

250ml/8 fl oz/1 cup groundnut (peanut) oil

30ml/2 tbsp fresh lemon juice

45ml/3 tbsp finely chopped spring
onions (scallions)

30ml/2 tbsp chopped drained capers

45ml/3 tbsp finely chopped sour dill pickles

45ml/3 tbsp finely chopped fresh parsley

1 In a bowl, beat the egg yolk with a wire whisk. Add the white wine vinegar and mustard and continue to whisk for about 10 seconds. Whisk the oil into the mixture in a slow, steady stream.

2 Add the lemon juice, spring onions, capers, sour dill pickles and parsley and mix well. Keep chilled; use within 2 days.

Energy 1662kcal/6835kJ; **Protein** 5.3g; **Carbohydrate** 2.7g, of which sugars 2.4g; **Fat** 181.2g, of which saturates 19.8g; **Cholesterol** 202mg; **Calcium** 141mg; **Fibre** 3.2g; **Sodium** 29mg.

Mint sauce

This sauce, with its tangy vinegar taste, is usually served with roast lamb.

INGREDIENTS

Makes about 300ml/^{1}/$_2$ pint/1^1/$_4$ cups

1 large bunch mint, finely chopped

105ml/7 tbsp boiling water

150ml/^{1}/$_4$ pint/^{2}/$_3$ cup wine vinegar

30ml/2 tbsp sugar

1 Place the chopped mint in a 600ml/1-pint/2^1/$_4$-cup jug (pitcher).

2 Pour the boiling water slowly into the jug, covering the mint, and then leave it to infuse for about 10 minutes.

3 When the mint infusion has cooled until it has reached a lukewarm temperature, stir in the wine vinegar and sugar.

4 Continue stirring (but do not mash up). Mint sauce will keep for up to 6 months stored in the refrigerator, but it is best used within 3 weeks.

Energy 161kcal/685kJ; **Protein** 3.9g; **Carbohydrate** 36.6g, of which sugars 31.3g; **Fat** 0.7g, of which saturates 0g; **Cholesterol** 0mg; **Calcium** 226mg; **Fibre** 0g; **Sodium** 17mg.

Horseradish sauce

This has a very strong flavour that complements steak or roast beef.

INGREDIENTS

Makes about 200ml/7fl oz/scant 1 cup

45ml/3 tbsp horseradish root

15ml/1 tbsp white wine vinegar

5ml/1 tsp sugar

pinch of salt

150ml/^{1}/$_4$ pint/^{2}/$_3$ cup thick double
(heavy) cream, for serving

1 Peel the horseradish root and grate it finely in a food processor. Horseradish is powerful, so submerge it in water while you peel it. Place the grated horseradish in a bowl, then wash your hands.

2 Add the white wine vinegar to the bowl, with the sugar and the salt. Stir until thoroughly combined.

3 Pour into a sterilized jar. It will keep in the refrigerator for 6 months. A few hours before serving the sauce, stir in the cream.

Energy 774kcal/3190kJ; **Protein** 2.8g; **Carbohydrate** 9.9g, of which sugars 9.8g; **Fat** 80.7g, of which saturates 50.1g; **Cholesterol** 206mg; **Calcium** 98mg; **Fibre** 1.1g; **Sodium** 40mg.

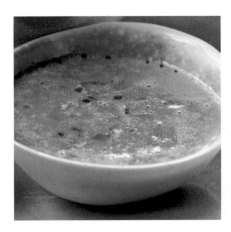

Beurre blanc

A reduction of white wine and vinegar forms the base for this rich sauce.

INGREDIENTS

Makes about 150ml/^{1}/4 pint/^{2}/3 cup
3 shallots, very finely chopped
45ml/3 tbsp dry white wine or court-bouillon
45ml/3 tbsp white wine vinegar or
  tarragon vinegar
115g/4oz/^{1}/2 cup chilled unsalted
  butter, diced
lemon juice (optional)
salt and ground white pepper

1 Put the shallots in a pan with the wine or court-bouillon and vinegar. Gently bring to the boil and cook over a high heat until only about 30ml/2 tbsp liquid remains in the pan.

2 Remove the pan from the heat and leave to cool until the reduced liquid is lukewarm.

3 Whisk in the butter, one piece at a time, to make a pale, creamy sauce. Taste, then season and add a little lemon juice to taste, if you like.

4 If you are not serving the sauce immediately, keep it warm in the top of a double boiler set over simmering water.

Energy 869kcal/3576kJ; **Protein** 1.3g; **Carbohydrate** 4.7g, of which sugars 3.4g; **Fat** 94.1g, of which saturates 62.1g; **Cholesterol** 265mg; **Calcium** 32mg; **Fibre** 0.8g; **Sodium** 39mg.

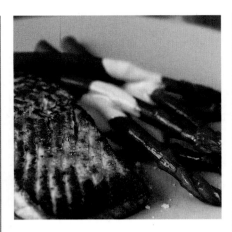

Hollandaise sauce

This is an essential part of Eggs Benedict, but is also delicious served on vegetables.

INGREDIENTS

Makes about 135ml/4fl oz/^{1}/₂ cup
115g/4oz/^{1}/2 cup unsalted butter
2 egg yolks
15–30ml/1–2 tbsp white wine vinegar or
  tarragon vinegar
salt and ground white pepper

1 Melt the butter in a small pan over a medium heat. Put the egg yolks and vinegar in a small bowl. Add salt and pepper and whisk until the mixture is completely smooth.

2 Slowly pour the melted butter in a steady stream on to the egg yolk mixture, beating vigorously the whole time with a wooden spoon to make a smooth, creamy sauce.

3 Taste the sauce and add more vinegar, and season, if necessary. Serve.

Cook's tip

Instead of adding the butter to the egg mixture in the bowl, you could put the mixture in a food processor and add the butter through the feeder tube, with the motor running.

Energy 874kcal/3596kJ; **Protein** 5.8g; **Carbohydrate** 0.6g, of which sugars 0.6g; **Fat** 94.3g, of which saturates 56.4g; **Cholesterol** 580mg; **Calcium** 60mg; **Fibre** 0g; **Sodium** 27mg.

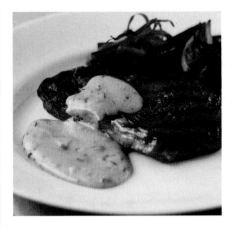

Béarnaise sauce

This rich buttery sauce is often served with 'steak frites' in France.

INGREDIENTS

Makes about 300ml/^{1}/2 pint/1^1/4 cups
90ml/6 tbsp white wine vinegar
12 black peppercorns
2 bay leaves
2 shallots, finely chopped
4 fresh tarragon sprigs
4 egg yolks
225g/8oz/1 cup unsalted butter, diced and
  warmed to room temperature
30ml/2 tbsp chopped fresh tarragon
salt and freshly ground white pepper

1 Put the white wine vinegar, peppercorns, bay leaves, shallots and tarragon sprigs in a pan and simmer until reduced to 30ml/2 tbsp. Strain through a fine sieve (strainer).

2 Beat the egg yolks with salt and ground white pepper in a heatproof bowl. Stand over a pan of gently simmering water, then beat the strained vinegar into the yolks.

3 Beat in the butter, one piece at a time. Beat the tarragon into the sauce and remove from the heat. It should be smooth, thick and glossy.

Energy 1919kcal/7900kJ; **Protein** 14.2g; **Carbohydrate** 1.4g, of which sugars 1.1g; **Fat** 206.4g, of which saturates 127.8g; **Cholesterol** 1324mg; **Calcium** 227mg; **Fibre** 2.5g; **Sodium** 1740mg.

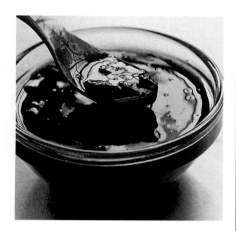

Sweet chilli sauce

This Thai sauce is great served as a dipping sauce with spring rolls.

INGREDIENTS

Makes about 350ml/12fl oz/1^{1}/$_{2}$ cups

6 large red chillies

60ml/4 tbsp rice vinegar or wine vinegar

250g/9oz caster (superfine) sugar

5ml/1 tsp salt

4 garlic cloves, chopped

10ml/2 tsp fish sauce

1 Cut the red chillies in half lengthways, then carefully remove the seeds with a sharp knife. Soak the seeds in hot water for about 15 minutes.

2 Chop the chilli flesh and place in a food processor. Drain the seeds and add them to the food processor. Add the vinegar, sugar, salt and garlic.

3 Blend in the food processor until the mixture is smooth, then transfer to a small pan and cook over a medium heat for about 20 minutes, or until the sauce has thickened.

4 Leave the sauce to cool, then stir in the fish sauce. The sweet chilli sauce can be stored in the refrigerator in an airtight container for 1–2 weeks.

Energy 1032kcal/4398kJ; Protein 6.7g; Carbohydrate 265.8g, of which sugars 262.4g; Fat 0.8g, of which saturates 0g; Cholesterol 0mg; Calcium 174mg; Fibre 0.8g; Sodium 2275mg.

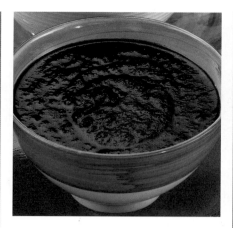

Chilli sauce

Serve this fiery sauce as a dip with raw vegetables or tortilla chips.

INGREDIENTS

Makes about 250ml/8fl oz/1 cup

15ml/1 tbsp olive oil

1 small onion, finely chopped

1 garlic clove, crushed

200g/7oz can chopped tomatoes

1 fresh red chilli, seeded and finely chopped

15ml/1 tbsp balsamic vinegar

15ml/1 tbsp chopped fresh
   coriander (cilantro), optional

salt and ground black pepper

1 Cook the onion and garlic in the oil for 5–10 minutes, or until soft.

2 Add the chopped tomatoes to the pan, with their juice. Stir in the chopped chilli and balsamic vinegar.

3 Cook gently for 10 minutes, or until the mixture has reduced and thickened.

4 Check the seasoning, and adjust if necessary. Stir in the chopped coriander, if using, and serve hot.

Cook's tip

If you like your chilli sauce really fiery, use two red chillies instead of one.

Energy 165kcal/684kJ; Protein 3.3g; Carbohydrate 11.5g, of which sugars 10.1g; Fat 12.1g, of which saturates 1.7g; Cholesterol 0mg; Calcium 67mg; Fibre 3.6g; Sodium 27mg.

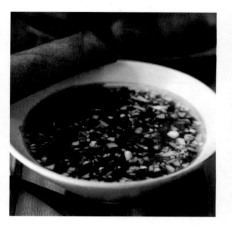

Coconut vinegar sauce

The main ingredient of coconut vinegar gives this sauce a real Filipino taste.

INGREDIENTS

Makes about 150ml/^{1}/$_{4}$ pint/^{2}/$_{3}$ cup

60–75ml/4–5 tbsp coconut vinegar

3 red chillies, seeded and finely chopped

4 spring onions (scallions), finely chopped

4 garlic cloves, finely chopped

Place all the ingredients together in a bowl and mix thoroughly. Spoon into a jar, cover and store in the refrigerator for up to 1 week.

Energy 41kcal/171kJ; Protein 4.1g; Carbohydrate 4.9g, of which sugars 1.9g; Fat 0.7g, of which saturates 0.1g; Cholesterol 0mg; Calcium 37mg; Fibre 1.4g; Sodium 8mg.

Redcurrant Sauce

Serve this quick and easy redcurrant sauce with roast meats.

INGREDIENTS

Makes about 150ml/^{1}/$_{4}$ pint/^{2}/$_{3}$ cup

115g/4oz/1 cup fresh or frozen redcurrants

10ml/2 tsp clear honey

5ml/1 tsp balsamic vinegar

30ml/2 tbsp finely chopped mint

Place all the ingredients in a bowl and mash them together with a fork. Store in the refrigerator and use within 2 days.

Energy 74kcal/316kJ; Protein 2.2g; Carbohydrate 16.8g, of which sugars 15.2g; Fat 0.2g, of which saturates 0g; Cholesterol 0mg; Calcium 133mg; Fibre 4.1g; Sodium 9mg.

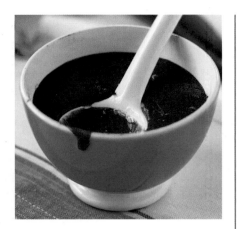

Mustard and dill sauce

This sauce is traditionally served with salmon gravadlax.

INGREDIENTS

Makes about 200ml/7fl oz/scant 1 cup

1 egg yolk

30ml/2 tbsp brown French mustard

2.5–5ml/^{1}/2–1 tsp soft dark brown sugar

15ml/1 tbsp white wine vinegar

90ml/6 tbsp sunflower or vegetable oil

30ml/2 tbsp finely chopped fresh dill

salt and ground black pepper

1 Put the egg yolk in a small bowl and add the mustard with a little soft brown sugar to taste. Beat with a wooden spoon until smooth.

2 Stir in the white wine vinegar, then whisk in the sunflower or vegetable oil, drop by drop to begin with.

3 As the sauce gets thicker, the oil can be poured in a steady stream. As the oil is added, the dressing will start to thicken and emulsify.

4 When all of the oil has been completely amalgamated into the sauce, season.

5 Stir in the chopped fresh dill. Cover and chill for 2 hours before serving.

Energy 716kcal/2950kJ; **Protein** 5.9g; **Carbohydrate** 6.3g, of which sugars 5.6g; **Fat** 74.3g, of which saturates 8.6g; **Cholesterol** 202mg; **Calcium** 106mg; **Fibre** 1.5g; **Sodium** 89mg.

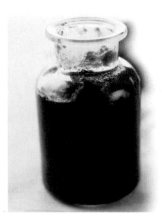

Barbecue sauce

This sauce will enliven burgers and other food cooked on the barbecue.

INGREDIENTS

Makes about 500ml/17fl oz/generous 2 cups

30ml/2 tbsp vegetable oil

1 large onion, chopped

2 garlic cloves, crushed

400g/14oz can tomatoes

30ml/2 tbsp Worcestershire sauce

15ml/1 tbsp white wine vinegar

45ml/3 tbsp honey

5ml/1 tsp mustard powder

2.5ml/^{1}/2 tsp chilli seasoning or mild chilli powder

salt and ground black pepper

1 In a large pan, heat the oil and fry the onion and garlic until soft. Stir in the remaining ingredients and gently bring to the boil.

2 Simmer the sauce, uncovered, for 15–20 minutes, stirring occasionally. Cool slightly. Pour the sauce into a food processor or blender and process until smooth.

3 Leave the sauce as it is, or press through a sieve (strainer) for a smoother result. Adjust the seasoning before serving. Store in the refrigerator and use within 2 weeks.

Energy 572kcal/2397kJ; **Protein** 9.1g; **Carbohydrate** 83.7g, of which sugars 73.6g; **Fat** 25.4g, of which saturates 2.7g; **Cholesterol** 0mg; **Calcium** 197mg; **Fibre** 9.6g; **Sodium** 413mg.

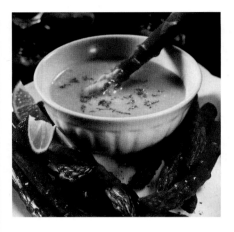

Lime butter sauce

Serve this creamy sauce as a dip for vegetables such as asparagus.

INGREDIENTS

Makes about 400ml/14fl oz/1^2/3 cups

90ml/6tbsp dry white wine

90ml/6 tbsp white wine vinegar

3 shallots, finely chopped

225g/8oz/1 cup very cold unsalted butter, diced

juice of 1 lime

salt and ground black pepper

lime wedges, to serve

1 Mix the wine and the vinegar in a stainless steel pan with the chopped shallots, and simmer until the liquid has reduced down to about 15ml/1 tbsp.

2 Remove the pan from the heat, then vigorously whisk in the butter until the sauce thickens.

3 Whisk in the lime juice until it is thoroughly combined. Taste the sauce and adjust the seasoning if necessary.

Cook's tip

Do not allow the sauce to boil. If the butter is taking a long time to melt, put the pan back over a gentle heat to speed up the process.

Energy 1739kcal/7156kJ; **Protein** 1.9g; **Carbohydrate** 5.3g, of which sugars 3.9g; **Fat** 183.9g, of which saturates 121.5g; **Cholesterol** 518mg; **Calcium** 57mg; **Fibre** 0.8g; **Sodium** 88mg.

VINEGAR IN SALADS

Shaken into dressings or drizzled over to taste, all sorts of vinegars can be used to complement all varieties of salad ingredients.

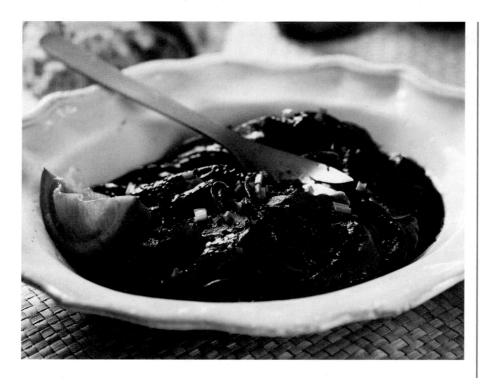

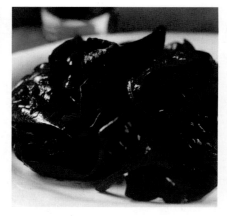

Anchovy and roasted pepper salad

The rich balsamic vinegar in this salad really brings out the flavour of the roasted peppers.

INGREDIENTS

Serves 4

2 red, 2 orange and 2 yellow (bell) peppers, halved and seeded

50g/2oz can anchovies in olive oil

2 garlic cloves

45ml/3 tbsp balsamic vinegar

salt and ground black pepper

1 Preheat the oven to 200°C/400°F/ Gas 6. Place the peppers, cut side down, in a roasting pan. Roast for 40 minutes, until the skins are charred. Transfer the peppers to a bowl, cover with clear film (plastic wrap) and leave for 15 minutes.

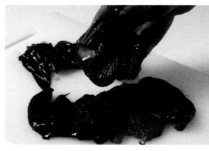

2 Peel the peppers, then cut them into chunky strips. Drain the anchovies, reserving the olive oil, and halve the fillets lengthways.

3 Slice the garlic as thinly as possible and place it in a large bowl. Stir in the olive oil, vinegar and a little pepper. Add the peppers and anchovies and use a spoon and fork to fold the ingredients together. Cover and chill until ready to serve.

Energy 108kcal/453kJ; **Protein** 6g; **Carbohydrate** 16.4g, of which sugars 15.5g; **Fat** 2.4g, of which saturates 0.5g; **Cholesterol** 8mg; **Calcium** 83mg; **Fibre** 4.6g; **Sodium** 506mg.

Warm chorizo and spinach salad

The ingredients in this salad are tossed in olive oil and sherry or wine vinegar.

INGREDIENTS

Serves 4

90ml/6 tbsp olive oil

225g/8oz baby spinach leaves

150g/5oz chorizo sausage, very thinly sliced

30ml/2 tbsp sherry vinegar or wine vinegar

salt and ground black pepper

1 Pour the oil into a large frying pan and add the sausage. Cook gently for about 3 minutes, until the sausage slices start to shrivel slightly and colour.

2 Discard any tough stalks from the spinach. Add the spinach leaves to the sausage and remove from the heat.

3 Toss the spinach in the warm oil until it just starts to wilt. Add the sherry or wine vinegar and a little seasoning.

4 Toss the ingredients together, then serve.

Energy 300kcal/1238kJ; **Protein** 5.6g; **Carbohydrate** 4.5g, of which sugars 1.4g; **Fat** 29g, of which saturates 7g; **Cholesterol** 18mg; **Calcium** 111mg; **Fibre** 1.4g; **Sodium** 364mg.

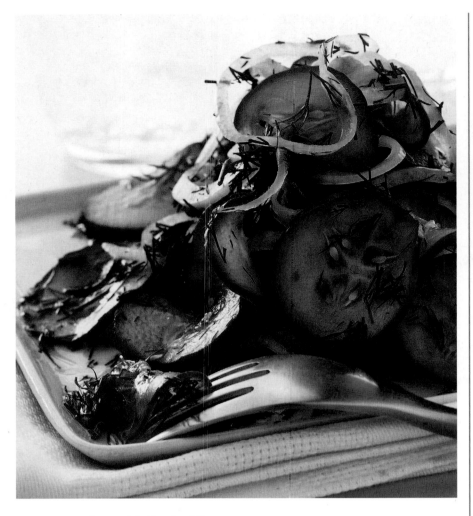

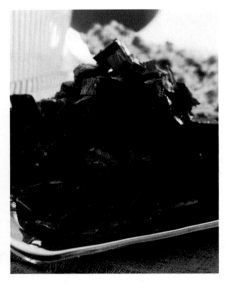

Sour cucumber with fresh dill

This is half pickle, half salad, and totally delicious served as a light meal or an appetizer. If possible, choose smooth-skinned, smallish cucumbers for this recipe as the larger ones tend to be less tender, with tough skins and bitter indigestible seeds.

INGREDIENTS

Serves 4

2 small cucumbers, thinly sliced

3 onions, thinly sliced

75–90ml/5–6 tbsp cider vinegar

30–45ml/2–3 tbsp chopped
  fresh dill

salt and ground black pepper

1 In a large mixing bowl, combine together the thinly sliced cucumbers and the thinly sliced onion.

2 Season the vegetables with salt and toss together until they are thoroughly combined. Leave the mixture to stand in a cool place for 5–10 minutes.

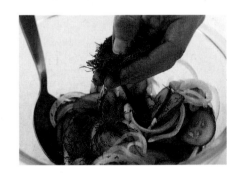

3 Add the cider vinegar, 30–45ml/2–3 tbsp water and the chopped fresh dill to the cucumber and onion mixture. Toss all the ingredients together until well combined, then chill in the refrigerator for a few hours, or until ready to serve.

Energy 89kcal/375kJ; **Protein** 2g; **Carbohydrate** 20.7g, of which sugars 18.3g; **Fat** 0.4g, of which saturates 0g; **Cholesterol** 0mg; **Calcium** 63mg; **Fibre** 2.3g; **Sodium** 9mg.

Beetroot with fresh mint

Balsamic vinegar is mixed with oil and mint and used as a marinade.

INGREDIENTS

Serves 4

4–6 cooked beetroot (beets)

15–30ml/1–2 tbsp balsamic vinegar

30ml/2 tbsp olive oil

1 bunch fresh mint, leaves stripped and
  thinly shredded

salt and ground black pepper

1 Slice the beetroot or cut into even-size dice with a sharp knife. Put the beetroot in a small bowl.

2 Add the balsamic vinegar, olive oil and a pinch of salt to the beetroot and toss together to combine.

3 Add half of the thinly shredded fresh mint to the salad and toss together lightly until thoroughly combined. Season to taste.

4 Place in the refrigerator and chill for about 1 hour. Serve the salad garnished with the remaining shredded mint leaves sprinkled over the top.

Energy 90kcal/378kJ; **Protein** 1.7g; **Carbohydrate** 8.9g, of which sugars 8.3g; **Fat** 5.6g, of which saturates 0.8g; **Cholesterol** 0mg; **Calcium** 21mg; **Fibre** 1.9g; **Sodium** 66mg.

VINEGAR IN FISH AND SHELLFISH DISHES

For marinating, poaching or dressing, vinegar has many classic and contemporary associations with fish and shellfish dishes.

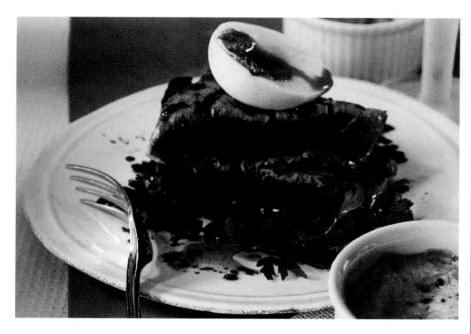

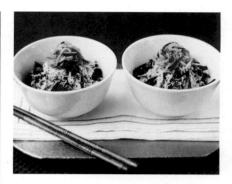

Japanese crab meat in vinegar

Rice vinegar is used widely in Japanese cooking – here as a dressing for crab.

INGREDIENTS

Serves 4

½ red (bell) pepper, seeded and sliced

pinch of salt

275g/10oz cooked white crab meat

about 300g/11oz cucumber, seeds removed

For the vinegar mixture

15ml/1 tbsp rice vinegar

10ml/2 tsp caster (superfine) sugar

10ml/2 tsp shoyu (soy sauce)

1 Sprinkle the pepper slices with salt and leave for 15 minutes. Rinse well and drain.

2 Combine the rice vinegar, sugar and shoyu in a bowl.

3 Loosen the crab meat and mix it with the pepper. Divide among four bowls.

4 Finely grate the cucumber. Mix the grated cucumber with the vinegar mixture, and pour a quarter into each bowl. Serve immediately.

Energy 82kcal/345kJ; **Protein** 13.3g; **Carbohydrate** 5.6g, of which sugars 5.4g; **Fat** 0.8g, of which saturates 0.1g; **Cholesterol** 50mg; **Calcium** 100mg; **Fibre** 0.9g; **Sodium** 560mg.

Seared tuna Niçoise

This simplified modern version of the traditional Tuna Niçoise is given a delicious aroma by the addition of sherry vinegar and garlic-infused oil. Serve with a green salad and fresh crusty bread.

INGREDIENTS

Serves 4

4 tuna steaks, about 150g/5oz each

45ml/3 tbsp garlic-infused olive oil

30ml/2 tbsp sherry vinegar or wine vinegar

2 eggs

salt and ground black pepper

1 Put the tuna steaks in a shallow non-metallic dish. Mix the oil and vinegar together and season with salt and pepper.

2 Pour the mixture over the tuna steaks and turn them to coat in the marinade. Cover and marinate for up to 1 hour.

3 Heat a griddle pan until smoking hot. Remove the tuna steaks from the marinade and lay them on the griddle pan. Cook for 2–3 minutes on each side, so that they are still pink in the centre. Remove from the pan and set aside.

4 Meanwhile, cook the eggs in a pan of boiling water for 5–6 minutes, then cool under cold running water. Shell the eggs and cut in half lengthways.

5 Pour the marinade on to the griddle pan and cook until it starts to bubble.

6 Divide the tuna steaks among four serving plates and top each with half an egg.

7 Drizzle the marinade over the top of the tuna and serve immediately.

Energy 578kcal/2408kJ; **Protein** 46.4g; **Carbohydrate** 15g, of which sugars 10.6g; **Fat** 37.5g, of which saturates 7.1g; **Cholesterol** 235mg; **Calcium** 127mg; **Fibre** 4.7g; **Sodium** 585mg.

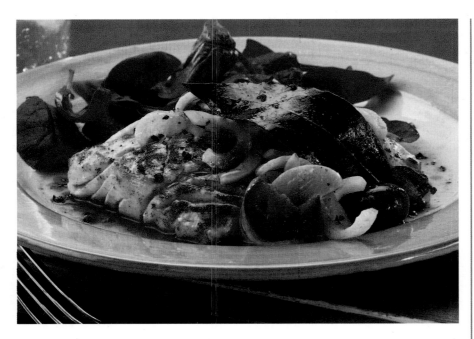

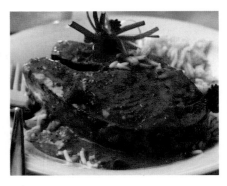

Coconut salmon

White wine vinegar forms the base of the spicy marinade for the salmon.

INGREDIENTS

Serves 4

10ml/2 tsp ground cumin

10ml/2 tsp chilli powder

2.5ml/^{1}/2 tsp ground turmeric

30ml/2 tbsp white wine vinegar

1.5ml/^{1}/4 tsp salt

4 salmon steaks, each about 175g/6oz

1 onion, chopped

2 fresh green chillies, seeded and chopped

2 garlic cloves, crushed

2.5cm/1in piece fresh root ginger, grated

45ml/3 tbsp vegetable oil

5ml/1 tsp ground coriander

175ml/6fl oz/^{3}/4 cup coconut milk

1 Mix 5ml/1 tsp of the ground cumin with the chilli powder, turmeric, vinegar and salt. Rub the paste over the salmon and marinate for 15 minutes.

2 Fry the onion, chillies, garlic and ginger in the oil for 5 minutes. Put into a food processor and process to a smooth paste.

3 Return the onion paste to the pan. Add the remaining cumin, the coriander and coconut milk. Bring to the boil and simmer for 5 minutes. Add the salmon steaks, cover and cook for 15 minutes, until tender. Serve with rice.

Energy 416kcal/1729kJ; **Protein** 36.2g; **Carbohydrate** 5.2g, of which sugars 4.8g; **Fat** 27.9g, of which saturates 4.4g; **Cholesterol** 88mg; **Calcium** 75mg; **Fibre** 1.1g; **Sodium** 132mg.

Escabeche

In this classic Mexican dish, the raw fish is initially marinated in lime juice, but is then cooked before being pickled in white wine vinegar.

INGREDIENTS

Serves 4

900g/2lb whole fish fillets

juice of 2 limes

300ml/^{1}/2 pint/1^1/4 cups olive oil

6 peppercorns

3 garlic cloves, sliced

2.5ml/^{1}/2 tsp ground cumin

2.5ml/^{1}/2 tsp dried oregano

2 bay leaves

50g/2oz/^{1}/3 cup pickled jalapeño chilli slices, chopped

1 onion, thinly sliced

250ml/8fl oz/1 cup white wine vinegar

150g/5oz/1^1/4 cups green olives stuffed with pimiento, to garnish

1 Place the fish fillets in a single layer in a shallow non-metallic dish.

2 Pour the lime juice over, turn the fillets over once to ensure that they are completely coated, then cover the dish and leave to marinate for about 15 minutes.

3 Drain the fish in a colander, then pat the fillets dry with kitchen paper. Heat 60ml/4 tbsp of the oil in a large frying pan, add the fish fillets and sauté for 5–6 minutes, turning once, until they are golden brown. Use a fish slice or metal spatula to transfer them to a shallow dish that will hold them in a single layer.

4 Heat 30ml/2 tbsp of the remaining oil in a frying pan. Add the peppercorns, garlic, ground cumin, oregano, bay leaves and jalapeños, and cook over a low heat for 2 minutes, then increase the heat, add the onion slices and vinegar and bring to the boil. Lower the heat and simmer for 4 minutes.

5 Remove the pan from the heat and carefully add the remaining oil. Stir well, then pour the mixture over the fish. Leave to cool, then cover the dish and marinate for 24 hours in the refrigerator.

6 When you are ready to serve, drain off the liquid and garnish the pickled fish with the stuffed olives. Salad leaves would make a good accompaniment.

Energy 414kcal/1720kJ; **Protein** 41.9g; **Carbohydrate** 1.3g, of which sugars 1g; **Fat** 26.7g, of which saturates 3.2g; **Cholesterol** 104mg; **Calcium** 30mg; **Fibre** 0.2g; **Sodium** 137mg.

VINEGAR IN POULTRY DISHES

Vinegar is very useful for marinating and dressing poultry and meat, but it is also invaluable in some recipes for braising or deglazing.

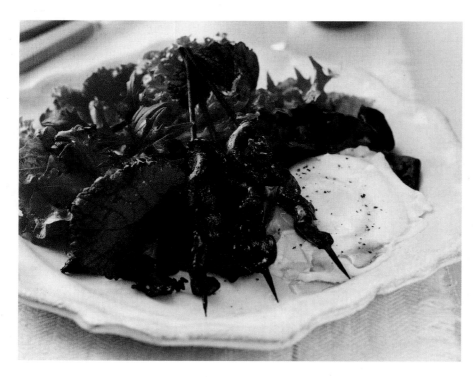

4 Grill (broil) for about 5 minutes, then turn the skewers and drizzle with the remaining oil. Grill for a further 3 minutes, or until the duck is cooked through and golden.

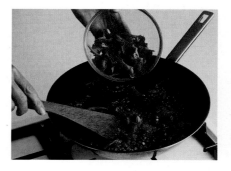

5 Meanwhile, melt the butter in a frying pan and cook the finely chopped shallot until softened. Add the chanterelle mushrooms and cook over a high heat for 5 minutes, stirring occasionally.

6 Poach the eggs while the chanterelles are cooking. Half fill a frying pan with water, add salt and heat until simmering. Break the eggs one at a time into a cup before tipping carefully into the water. Poach the eggs gently for 3 minutes, or until the whites are set. Use a draining spoon to transfer the eggs to a warm plate and trim off any untidy white.

7 Arrange the salad leaves on serving plates, then add the chanterelles and duck.

8 Carefully add the poached eggs. Drizzle with olive oil and season with ground black pepper.

Energy 271kcal/1132kJ; **Protein** 29.2g; **Carbohydrate** 1.5g, of which sugars 1.1g; **Fat** 18.6g, of which saturates 3.9g; **Cholesterol** 314mg; **Calcium** 51mg; **Fibre** 0.7g; **Sodium** 196mg.

Warm duck salad with poached eggs

This salad looks spectacular and tastes divine, and makes a perfect celebration starter or, accompanied by warm crusty bread, a light lunch or supper dish. The duck is marinated in a soy sauce and vinegar mixture.

INGREDIENTS

Serves 4

3 skinless, boneless duck breasts, thinly sliced

30ml/2 tbsp soy sauce

30ml/2 tbsp balsamic vinegar

30ml/2 tbsp groundnut (peanut) oil

25g/1oz/2 tbsp unsalted butter

1 shallot, finely chopped

115g/4oz/1½ cups chanterelle mushrooms

4 eggs

50g/2oz mixed salad leaves

salt and ground black pepper

30ml/2 tbsp extra virgin olive oil, to serve

1 Toss the duck in the soy sauce and balsamic vinegar. Cover and chill for 30 minutes to allow the duck to infuse in the soy sauce and vinegar.

2 Meanwhile, Soak 12 bamboo skewers (about 13cm/5in long) in water to prevent them from burning during cooking. Preheat the grill (broiler) to medium.

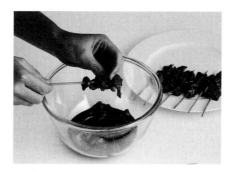

3 Thread the duck on to the skewers, pleating them neatly. Place on a grill pan and drizzle with half the oil.

Adobo chicken and pork cooked with vinegar and ginger

This Filipino dish can also be prepared with fish, shellfish and vegetables. Use coconut vinegar for an authentic flavour, or white wine vinegar if it is unavailable.

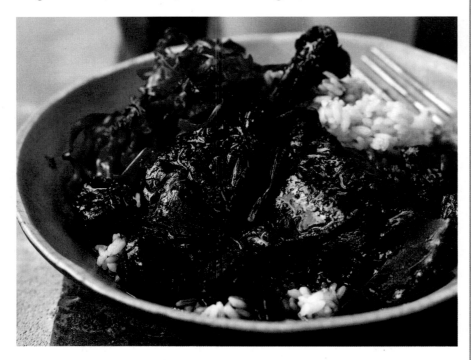

INGREDIENTS

Serves 4–6

30ml/2 tbsp coconut oil

6–8 garlic cloves, crushed whole

50g/2oz fresh root ginger, sliced
    into matchsticks

6 spring onions (scallions), cut into
    2.5cm/1in pieces

5–10ml/1–2 tsp whole black
    peppercorns, crushed

30ml/2 tbsp palm sugar (jaggery) or
    muscovado sugar

8–10 chicken thighs, or thighs and drumsticks

350g/12 oz pork fillet (tenderloin),
    cut into chunks

150ml/^{1}/4 pint/^{2}/3 cup coconut vinegar

150ml/^{1}/4 pint/^{2}/3 cup dark soy sauce

300ml/^{1}/2 pint/1^1/4 cups chicken stock

2–3 bay leaves

salt

stir-fried greens and cooked rice, to serve

1 Heat the oil in a wok, stir in the garlic and ginger and fry until fragrant and beginning to colour. Add the spring onions and black pepper and stir in the sugar.

2 Add the chicken and pork to the wok and fry until they begin to colour.

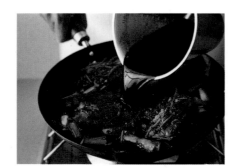

3 Pour in the vinegar, soy sauce and chicken stock and add the bay leaves.

4 Bring to the boil, reduce the heat, and cover. Simmer gently for 1 hour, until the meat is tender and the liquid has reduced.

5 Season the stew with salt to taste and serve with stir-fried greens and rice, over which the cooking liquid is spooned.

Energy 270kcal/1135kJ; **Protein** 42.2g; **Carbohydrate** 9g, of which sugars 7.6g; **Fat** 7.4g, of which saturates 1.6g; **Cholesterol** 118mg; **Calcium** 24mg; **Fibre** 0.6g; **Sodium** 1892mg.

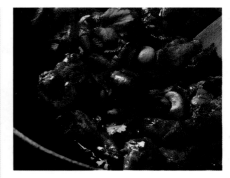

Sichuan chicken in kung po sauce

This is a classic Chinese dish.

INGREDIENTS

Serves 3

1 egg white

10ml/2 tsp cornflour (cornstarch)

2.5ml/^{1}/2 tsp salt

2 chicken breasts, cut into small pieces

10ml/2 tbsp yellow salted beans

15ml/1 tbsp hoisin sauce

5ml/1 tsp light brown sugar

15ml/1 tbsp rice wine

15ml/1 tbsp white wine vinegar

4 garlic cloves, crushed

150ml/^{1}/4 pint/^{2}/3 cup chicken stock

45ml/3 tbsp groundnut (peanut) oil

2–3 dried chillies, broken into small pieces

115g/4oz roasted cashew nuts

fresh coriander (cilantro) to garnish

1 Whisk the egg white, add the cornflour and salt, then stir in the chicken.

2 In a bowl, mash the beans. Stir in the hoisin sauce, sugar, rice wine, vinegar, garlic and stock.

3 In a wok, fry the chicken in the oil for 2 minutes, then drain over a bowl to collect the oil. Fry the chilli pieces in the reserved oil for 1 minute. Return the chicken to the wok with the bean sauce mixture. Bring to the boil, stir in the cashew nuts and serve garnished with coriander.

Energy 490kcal/2040kJ; **Protein** 37.7g; **Carbohydrate** 12.4g, of which sugars 2.6g; **Fat** 31.9g, of which saturates 5.6g; **Cholesterol** 82mg; **Calcium** 24mg; **Fibre** 1.9g; **Sodium** 204mg.

VINEGAR IN MEAT DISHES

Used in marinades or cooking sauces, vinegar can be used to make meat tender and moist, with rich sweet-sour flavours as a finishing touch.

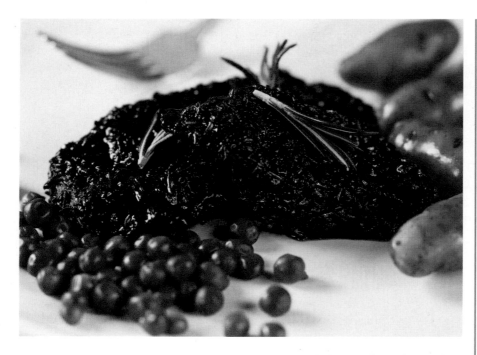

Lamb steaks with redcurrant vinegar glaze

This classic, simple dish is an excellent, quick recipe for cooking on the barbecue. The tangy flavour of redcurrants is a traditional accompaniment to lamb.

INGREDIENTS

Serves 4

4 large fresh rosemary sprigs

4 lamb leg steaks

75ml/5 tbsp redcurrant jelly

30ml/2 tbsp raspberry or red wine vinegar

salt and ground black pepper

1 Reserve the tips of the rosemary and chop the remaining leaves. Rub the chopped rosemary, salt and pepper all over the lamb.

2 Preheat the grill (broiler). Heat the redcurrant jelly gently in a small pan with 30ml/2 tbsp water. Stir in the vinegar.

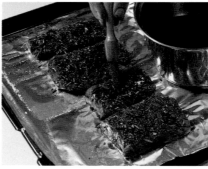

3 Place the steaks on a foil-lined grill (broiler) rack and brush with a little of the redcurrant glaze. Cook for 5 minutes on each side, until deep golden, brushing with more glaze.

4 Transfer the lamb to warmed plates. Tip any juices from the foil into the remaining glaze and heat through. Pour over the lamb and serve, garnished with the reserved rosemary.

Energy 301kcal/1,258kJ; **Protein** 24g; **Carbohydrate** 12g, of which sugars 12g; **Fat** 17g, of which saturates 8g; **Cholesterol** 94mg; **Calcium** 10mg; **Fibre** 0.0g; **Sodium** 100mg.

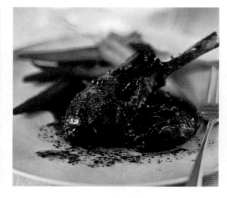

Sweet-and-sour lamb

Tender lamb chops are marinated, then cooked in balsamic vinegar.

INGREDIENTS

Serves 4

8 French-trimmed lamb loin chops

90ml/6 tbsp balsamic vinegar

30ml/2 tbsp caster (superfine) sugar

30ml/2 tbsp olive oil

salt and ground black pepper

1 Put the lamb chops in a shallow, non-metallic dish and drizzle over the balsamic vinegar. Sprinkle with sugar and season with salt and black pepper. Turn the chops to coat, cover with clear film (plastic wrap) and marinate for 20 minutes.

2 Heat the oil in a large frying pan and add the chops, reserving the marinade. Cook for 3–4 minutes on each side.

3 Pour the marinade into the pan and leave to bubble for about 2 minutes, or until reduced slightly. Remove from the pan and serve immediately.

Energy 258kcal/1077kJ; **Protein** 19.6g; **Carbohydrate** 7.9g, of which sugars 7.9g; **Fat** 16.7g, of which saturates 6g; **Cholesterol** 76mg; **Calcium** 12mg; **Fibre** 0g; **Sodium** 87mg.

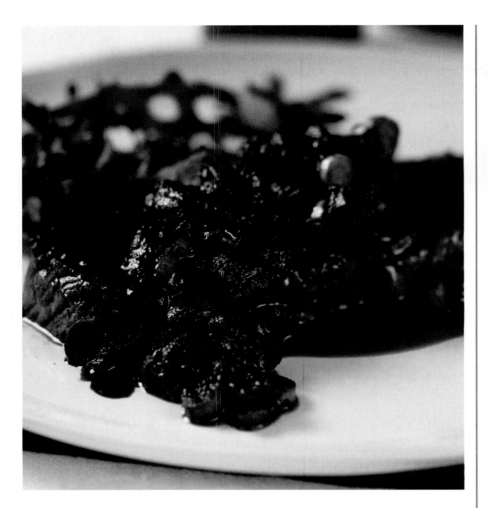

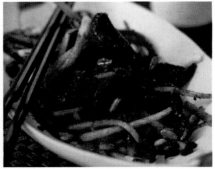

Beef with Asian pear

Rice vinegar is used to marinate the pear.

INGREDIENTS

Serves 4

300g/11oz fillet steak, thinly sliced

15ml/1 tbsp dark soy sauce

1 garlic clove, crushed

10ml/2 tsp sesame oil

1 Asian pear

15ml/1 tbsp sugar

15ml/1 tbsp rice vinegar

vegetable oil, for cooking

30ml/2 tbsp pine nuts

5 cooked chestnuts, finely chopped

salt and ground black pepper

1 Mix the steak with the soy sauce, garlic, sesame oil and a little salt and pepper and marinate for 20 minutes.

2 Meanwhile, peel, core and slice the pear, then cut the slices into fine strips. Place in a small bowl and pour in cold water to cover. Stir the sugar and rice vinegar into the bowl. Leave to stand for 5 minutes, then drain and set aside.

3 Heat a frying pan over a high heat and add a little vegetable oil. Add the beef with its marinade and sauté briefly, then reduce the heat and fry gently until the meat is well cooked. Transfer to a serving dish. Add the pear, pine nuts and chestnuts, toss together and serve.

Energy 234kcal/976kJ; **Protein** 18.6g; **Carbohydrate** 8.9g, of which sugars 5.2g; **Fat** 14g, of which saturates 3.5g; **Cholesterol** 44mg; **Calcium** 15mg; **Fibre** 1.5g; **Sodium** 300mg.

Steak with warm tomato salsa

A refreshing, tangy salsa of tomatoes, spring onions and balsamic vinegar makes a colourful topping for chunky, pan-fried steaks. Serve with potato wedges and a mixed leaf salad with a mustard dressing.

INGREDIENTS

Serves 4

2 steaks, about 2cm/3/4 in thick

4 large plum tomatoes

2 spring onions (scallions)

30ml/2 tbsp balsamic vinegar

salt and ground black pepper

1 Trim any excess fat from the steaks, then season on both sides with salt and pepper.

2 Heat a non-stick frying pan and cook the steaks for 3 minutes on each side for medium rare, or longer if you prefer.

3 Meanwhile, put the tomatoes in a heatproof bowl, cover with boiling water and leave for 1–2 minutes, until the skins start to split.

4 Drain and peel the tomatoes, then halve them and scoop out the seeds. Dice the tomato flesh. Thinly slice the spring onions.

5 Transfer the steaks to plates and keep warm.

6 Add the vegetables, balsamic vinegar, 30ml/2 tbsp water and a little seasoning to the cooking juices in the pan and stir briefly until warm, scraping up any meat residue. Spoon the salsa over the steaks to serve.

Energy 291kcal/1215kJ; **Protein** 35.3g; **Carbohydrate** 5g, of which sugars 5g; **Fat** 14.5g, of which saturates 5.9g; **Cholesterol** 87mg; **Calcium** 22mg; **Fibre** 1.7g; **Sodium** 110mg.

VINEGAR IN BAKING

It may seem surprising, but vinegar is a useful ingredient for baking many sweet dishes. Use to balance the sweetness of tarts and ensure cakes rise beautifully.

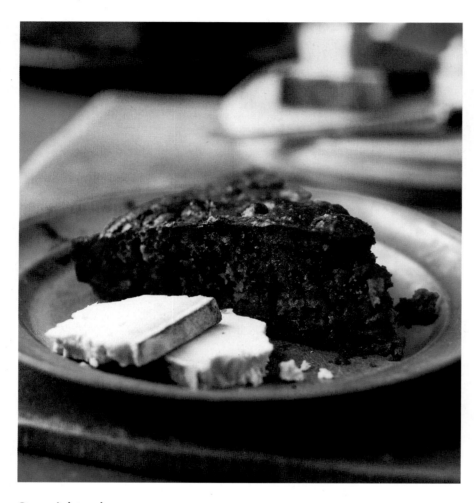

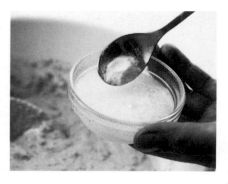

2 Mix the bicarbonate of soda with the vinegar and, as it froths, quickly stir it into the mixture. Cover the bowl and leave at room temperature for 8 hours.

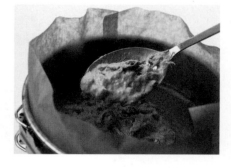

3 Preheat the oven to 180°C/360°F/ Gas 4. Grease a shallow 23cm/9 in round cake tin (pan) and line its base with baking parchment. Spoon the mixture into the prepared tin and level the top.

Overnight cake

Baking powder is a mixture of an acid and an alkali. When combined with moisture and heated, this mixture gives off carbon dioxide, which creates bubbles in a mixture and makes it rise. Cooking sets the mixture and traps the bubbles. Using vinegar, an acid, in the same mixture as bicarbonate of soda, an alkali, has the same effect. The following is a traditional British recipe for an eggless fruit cake. The vinegar will lose its acidity once the cake is cooked, providing just a hint of sharpness.

INGREDIENTS

Serves 4

225g/8oz/2 cups plain (all-purpose) flour

5ml/1 tsp ground cinnamon

5ml/1 tsp ground ginger

115g/4oz/^{1}/2 cup butter, diced

115g/4oz/^{2}/3 cup mixed dried fruit

300ml/^{1}/2 pint/1^1/4 cups milk

2.5ml/1/2 tsp bicarbonate of soda (baking soda)

15ml/1 tbsp cider vinegar or white vinegar

1 Sift the flour and spices together. Add the butter and rub in until the mixture resembles fine breadcrumbs. Stir in the dried fruit and enough milk to make a soft mix.

4 Put into the oven and cook for 1 hour or until firm to the touch and cooked through – a skewer inserted in the centre should come out clean. If the top starts to get too brown, cover with baking parchment.

5 Cool in the tin for 20 minutes, turn out and cool completely on a wire rack.

Energy 2069kcal/8681kJ; **Protein** 34.7g; **Carbohydrate** 267.9g, of which sugars 96.5g; **Fat** 103g, of which saturates 63.6g; **Cholesterol** 263mg; **Calcium** 780mg; **Fibre** 9.5g; **Sodium** 888mg.

Pavlova

There are three main elements that make pavlova different from other meringues: the addition of cornflour and vinegar; folding in, rather than whisking in, the sugar; and the depth of the cooked meringue. These differences help to create the soft, chewy centre.

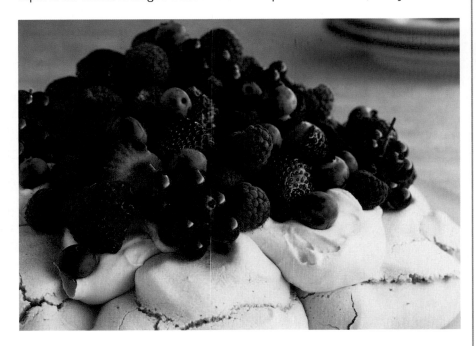

INGREDIENTS

Serves 4–6

4 egg whites

220g/7oz sugar

15–30ml/1–2 tbsp cornflour (cornstarch)

15ml/1 tbsp white wine vinegar

300ml/^{1}/$_2$ pint/1^1/$_2$ cups whipped cream

450g/1lb/4 cups mixed berries

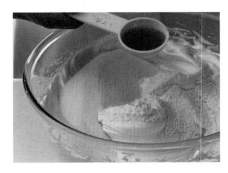

1 Whisk the egg whites to form soft peaks. Whisk in most of the sugar, reserving a small amount. Sift the cornflour over the meringue, then fold in the remaining sugar. Add the vinegar.

2 Fold in the vinegar with a large metal spoon until blended. Work gently to avoid knocking the air from the meringue.

3 Preheat the oven to 140°C/275°F/ Gas 1. Prepare a baking sheet, drawing a 23cm/9in circle in heavy pencil on the reverse of the paper.

4 Spread half the mixture into a thick, flat neat round, then spoon the rest in high swirls around the edge to create a border. Bake for 1–1^1/$_2$ hours until the meringue is firm, checking frequently.

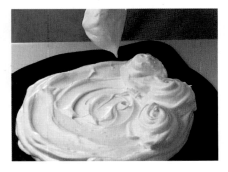

5 When cooked and cooled, peel off the paper and fill the pavlova shell with the whipped cream and the berries.

Energy 565kcal/2368kJ; **Protein** 5.6g; **Carbohydrate** 73.5g, of which sugars 66.6g; **Fat** 29.7g, of which saturates 18.5g; **Cholesterol** 78.8mg; **Calcium** 96.5mg; **Fibre** 1.3g; **Sodium** 104.8mg.

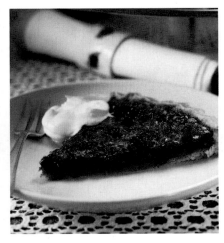

Currant and walnut tart

Add a little white wine vinegar to this tart to counter the sweetness.

INGREDIENTS

Serves 4

250g/9oz sweet pastry

1 egg

75g/3oz/scant ^{1}/$_2$ cup soft light brown sugar

50g/2oz/^{1}/$_4$ cup butter, melted

10ml/2 tsp white wine vinegar

115g/4oz/^{1}/$_2$ cup currants

25g/1oz/^{1}/$_4$ cup chopped walnuts

double (heavy) cream, to serve (optional)

1 Line a 20cm/8in flan tin (tart pan) with sweet pastry. Preheat the oven to 190°C/ 375°F/Gas 5.

2 Mix the egg, sugar and melted butter together. Stir the vinegar, currants and walnuts into the mixture.

3 Pour the mixture into the pastry case and bake for 30 minutes. Remove from the oven when thoroughly cooked, take out of the flan tin and leave to cool on a wire rack for at least 30 minutes.

4 Serve the tart on its own or with a dollop of fresh cream, if using.

Energy 312kcal/1,307kJ; **Protein** 3.4g; **Carbohydrate** 41.1g, of which sugars 41g; **Fat** 16.1g, of which saturates 7.3g; **Cholesterol** 74mg; **Calcium** 54mg; **Fibre** 0.8g; **Sodium** 99mg.

VINEGAR IN DRINKS

A little vinegar in sparkling mineral water makes a refreshing drink and an excellent alternative to an alcoholic drink or glass of wine. It is also used to give an edge to some cocktails.

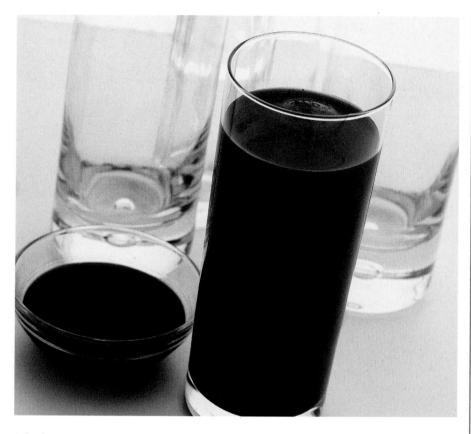

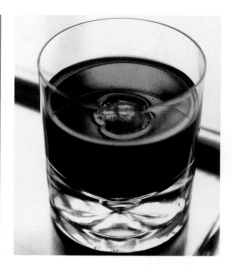

Prairie oyster

This cocktail, containing a dash of white wine vinegar, is said to cure hangovers.

INGREDIENTS

Makes about 45ml/3 tbsp

1 measure/1^1/$_2$ tbsp sweet (malmsey)
   Madeira, or cognac

^{1}/$_2$ measure/1 tsp white wine vinegar

^{1}/$_2$ measure/1 tsp Worcestershire sauce

pinch cayenne pepper

dash Tabasco

1 egg yolk

1 Add the Madeira or cognac, white wine vinegar, Worcestershire sauce, cayenne pepper and Tabasco to a small tumbler.

2 Mix well without ice, and then spoon the yolk very gently on top.

3 The preparation should then be swallowed in one gulp, without breaking the egg yolk.

Energy 112kcal/463kJ; **Protein** 3g; **Carbohydrate** 0.8g, of which sugars 0.7g; **Fat** 5.5g, of which saturates 1.6g; **Cholesterol** 202mg; **Calcium** 33mg; **Fibre** 0g; **Sodium** 69mg.

Virgin prairie oyster

This delicious non-alcoholic version of the classic hangover cure will help you to avoid hangovers altogether.

INGREDIENTS

Makes about 200ml/7fl oz/scant 1 cup

175ml/6fl oz tomato juice

^{1}/$_2$ measure/2 tsp Worcestershire sauce

^{1}/$_4$–^{1}/$_2$ measure/1–2 tsp balsamic vinegar

1 egg yolk

cayenne pepper, to taste

1 Measure the tomato juice into a large bar glass and stir over plenty of ice until well chilled.

2 Strain into a tall tumbler half-filled with ice cubes.

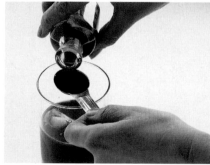

3 Add the Worcestershire sauce and balsamic vinegar to taste and mix with a swizzle-stick.

4 Carefully float the egg yolk on top of the drink and lightly dust with cayenne pepper.

Energy 92kcal/388kJ; **Protein** 4.4g; **Carbohydrate** 6.8g, of which sugars 6.7g; **Fat** 5.5g, of which saturates 1.6g; **Cholesterol** 202mg; **Calcium** 60mg; **Fibre** 1.1g; **Sodium** 532mg.

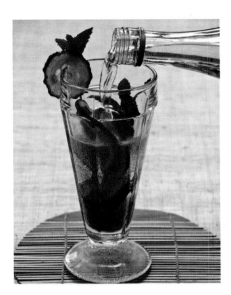

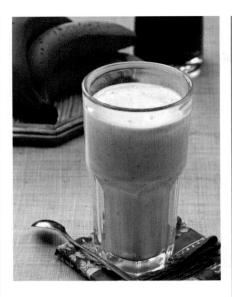

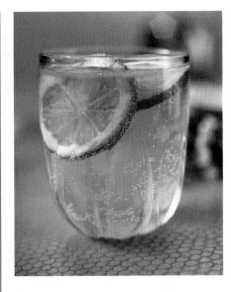

Vinegar spritzers

Mixing a little vinegar with mineral water makes a surprisingly tasty summer drink.

INGREDIENTS

Makes one glass

10ml/2 tsp fruit vinegar, such as raspberry, fig or blackberry

slices of cucumber, orange and apple

sprig of fresh mint

sparkling mineral water

1 Pour the fruit vinegar into a glass.

2 Add the slices of cucumber, orange and apple with a sprig of fresh mint and top up with sparkling mineral water.

Variations

Place 10ml/2 tsp raspberry vinegar in a glass and top up with sparkling water.

Sweet moscatel vinegar is fabulous in mineral water. Pour about 10ml/2 tsp in a wine glass and top up with still water.

Add balsamic vinegar to sparkling mineral water, allowing about 5ml/ 1 tsp per glass. This is similar to water with Angostura bitters.

Energy 24kcal/104kJ; Protein 0.3g; Carbohydrate 6.1g, of which sugars 6.1g; Fat 0.1g, of which saturates 0g; Cholesterol 0mg; Calcium 5mg; Fibre 1.1g; Sodium 4mg.

Vinegar smoothies

Adding vinegar to fruit smoothies gives them a tangy kick.

INGREDIENTS

Makes about 400ml/³/4 pint/scant 2 cups

15ml/1 tbsp fruit vinegar, such as raspberry, orange or blackberry

300ml/¹/2 pint/1¹/4 cup natural (plain) yogurt

fruit juice, such as apple

1 Pour the yogurt into a tall glass and add the fruit vinegar.

2 Top up the glass with fruit juice.

Variations

Try adding 10ml/2 tsp fermented fig vinegar for a rich, sweet-sour, caramel-fig flavoured drink.

Fruit vinegars such as raspberry, strawberry or blackberry are very good with banana or apple in smoothies, adding a pleasing sharpness.

Combine raspberry vinegar, honey and yogurt for a invigorating smoothie. Stir in a little raspberry and cranberry juice to thin the drink if necessary.

Energy 204kcal/861kJ; Protein 15.7g; Carbohydrate 31.5g, of which sugars 31.5g; Fat 3.1g, of which saturates 1.5g; Cholesterol 4mg; Calcium 576mg; Fibre 1.6g; Sodium 254mg.

Sparkling elderflower drink

This refreshing drink will keep in airtight bottles for up to a month.

INGREDIENTS

Makes 9.5 litres/2 gallons/2.4 US gallons

24 elderflower heads

2 lemons

1.3kg/3lb/scant 7 cups granulated (white) sugar

30ml/2 tbsp white wine vinegar or cider vinegar

9 litres/2 gallons/2.4 US gallons water

1 Find a clean bucket that you can cover with a clean cloth. Put all the ingredients into it.

2 Cover the bucket with a plastic sheet and leave overnight.

3 Strain the elderflower drink then pour into bottles, leaving a space of about 2.5cm/1in at the top.

4 Seal the bottles and leave for 2 weeks in a cool place. A fermentation takes place and the result is a delightful, sparkling, refreshing, non-alcoholic drink. Serve chilled with slices of lemon.

Energy 186kcal/793kJ; Protein 7.5g; Carbohydrate 34.6g, of which sugars 16.4g; Fat 3.1g, of which saturates 0.4g; Cholesterol 1mg; Calcium 137mg; Fibre 5.5g; Sodium 51mg.

VINEGAR IN PICKLES

Pickles can be sharp or sweet or a combination of the two. They are usually made by preserving raw or lightly cooked fruit or vegetables in spiced vinegar.

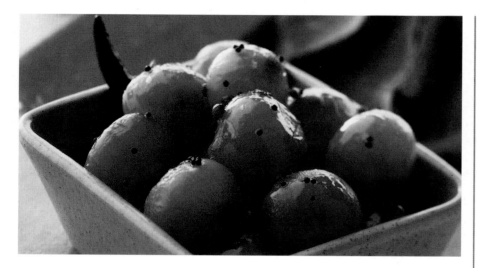

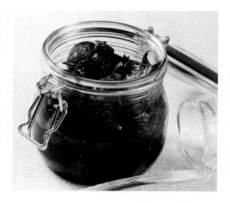

Shallots in balsamic vinegar

Whole shallots cooked in balsamic vinegar and herbs have a gentle taste.

Pickled onions

These powerful pickles should be made with malt vinegar and stored for at least 6 weeks before eating.

INGREDIENTS

Makes about 4 jars

1kg/2¼lb pickling onions, peeled

115g/4oz/½ cup salt

750ml/11/4 pints/3 cups malt vinegar

15ml/1 tbsp sugar

2–3 dried red chillies

5ml/1 tsp brown mustard seeds

15ml/1 tbsp coriander seeds

5ml/1 tsp allspice berries

5ml/1 tsp black peppercorns

5cm/2in piece fresh root ginger, sliced

2–3 blades mace

2–3 fresh bay leaves

1 Place the peeled onions in a bowl, cover with cold water, then drain the water into a pan.

2 Add the salt and heat slightly to dissolve, then cool before pouring the brine over the onions.

3 Place a plate inside the top of the bowl and weigh it down slightly so that it keeps all the onions submerged in the brine. Leave to stand for 24 hours.

4 Meanwhile, place the vinegar in a large pan. Wrap all the remaining ingredients, except the bay leaves, in a piece of muslin (cheesecloth). Bring to the boil, simmer for about 5 minutes, then remove the pan from the heat. Set aside and leave to infuse overnight.

5 The next day, drain the onions, rinse and pat dry. Pack them into sterilized 450g/1lb jars. Add some or all of the spice from the vinegar, except the ginger. The pickle will become hotter if you add the chillies. Pour the vinegar over to cover and add the bay leaves.

6 Seal the jars with non-metallic lids and store in a cool, dark place for at least 6 weeks before eating.

Energy 669kcal/2,775kJ; **Protein** 48.7g; **Carbohydrate** 5g, of which sugars 3.8g; **Fat** 45.9g, of which saturates 11.1g; **Cholesterol** 250mg; **Calcium** 37mg; **Fibre** 0.9g; **Sodium** 196mg.

INGREDIENTS

Makes 1 large jar

500g/1¼lb shallots

30ml/2 tbsp muscovado (molasses) sugar

fresh thyme sprigs

300ml/½ pint/1¼ cups balsamic vinegar

1 Put the unpeeled shallots in a bowl. Pour over boiling water and leave to stand for 2 minutes to loosen the skins. Drain and peel the shallots, leaving whole.

2 Put the sugar, thyme and vinegar in a pan and bring to the boil.

3 Add the shallots, cover and simmer gently for 40 minutes, or until the shallots are just tender.

4 Transfer to a warmed sterilized jar, packing the shallots down well. Seal and label the jar, then store in a cool, dark place for about 1 month before eating.

Energy 298kcal/1254kJ; **Protein** 6.1g; **Carbohydrate** 70.9g, of which sugars 59.3g; **Fat** 1g, of which saturates 0g; **Cholesterol** 0mg; **Calcium** 141mg; **Fibre** 7g; **Sodium** 17mg.

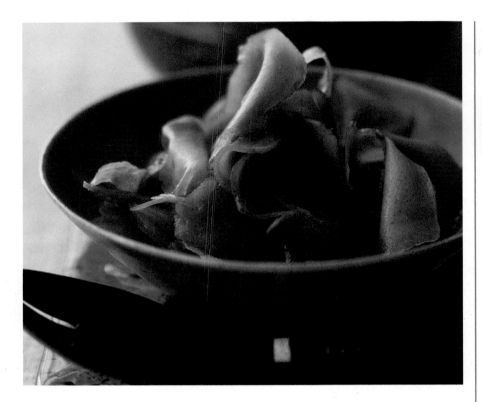

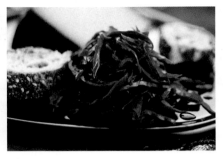

Pickled red cabbage

This delicately spiced and vibrant pickle
is made with red wine vinegar.

INGREDIENTS

Serves 4

675g/1^1/2lb/6 cups red cabbage, shredded

1 large Spanish (Bermuda) onion, sliced

30ml/2 tbsp sea salt

600ml/1 pint/2^1/2 cups red wine vinegar

75g/3oz/6 tbsp light muscovado
   (brown) sugar

15ml/1 tbsp coriander seeds

3 cloves

2.5cm/1in piece fresh root ginger

1 whole star anise

2 bay leaves

4 eating apples

1 Put the cabbage and onion in a bowl,
add the salt and mix well. Transfer the
mixture into a colander over a bowl and
leave to drain overnight.

2 The next day, rinse the vegetables,
drain and pat dry using kitchen paper.
Pour the vinegar into a pan, add the
sugar, spices and bay leaves and bring to
the boil. Remove from the heat and cool.

3 Core and chop the apples, then layer
with the cabbage and onions in
sterilized preserving jars. Pour over the
cooled spiced vinegar. Seal and store
for 1 week before eating. Eat within
2 months. Once opened, keep chilled.

Energy 674kcal/2868kJ; **Protein** 12g; **Carbohydrate**
161.4g, of which sugars 159.3g; **Fat** 2g, of which
saturates 0g; **Cholesterol** 0mg; **Calcium** 405mg; **Fibre**
23g; **Sodium** 64mg.

Pickled ginger

Warming, good for the heart,
and believed to aid digestion, ginger
finds its way into oriental cooking in
many dishes from salads, soups and
stir-fries to puddings. Chinese in origin,
ginger pickled in rice vinegar is often
served as a condiment with broths,
noodles and rice.

INGREDIENTS

Serves 4–6

225g/8oz fresh young ginger, peeled

10ml/2 tsp salt

200ml/7fl oz/1 cup white rice vinegar

50g/2oz/^{1}/4 cup sugar

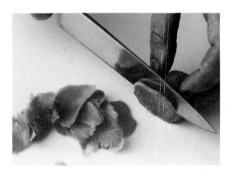

1 Place the ginger in a bowl and sprinkle
with salt. Cover and place in the
refrigerator for at least 24 hours.

2 Drain off any excess liquid and
pat the ginger dry with a clean dish
towel. Slice each knob of ginger very
finely along the grain, like thin rose
petals, and place them in a
clean bowl or a sterilized jar suitable
for storing.

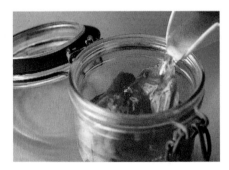

3 In a small bowl, beat the vinegar
and 50ml/2fl oz/1/4 cup cold water
with the sugar, until it has all
completely dissolved.

4 Pour the pickling liquid over the
ginger and cover or seal. Store in
the refrigerator or a cool place for
about 1 week.

Energy 36kcal/151kJ; **Protein** 0.2g; **Carbohydrate**
9.1g, of which sugars 9.1g; **Fat** 0.1g, of which saturates
0g; **Cholesterol** 0mg; **Calcium** 20mg; **Fibre** 0.4g;
Sodium 678mg.

VINEGAR IN RELISHES AND CHUTNEYS

Chutneys and relishes are made from finely cut ingredients, cooked with vinegar, a sweetener and frequently spices to make a thick, savoury jam-like mixture.

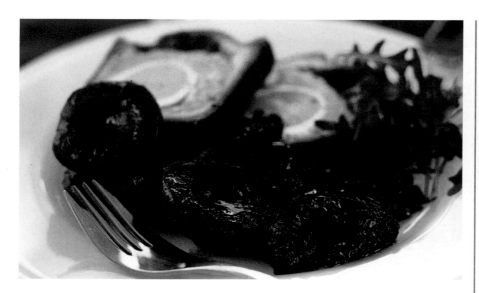

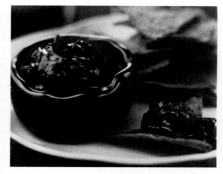

Tart tomato relish

Adding lime to this relish gives it a wonderfully tart, tangy flavour.

INGREDIENTS

Makes about 500g/1^{1}/4lb

2 pieces preserved stem ginger

1 lime

450g/1lb cherry tomatoes

115g/4oz/^{1}/2 cup muscovado (molasses) sugar

120ml/4fl oz/^{1}/2 cup white wine vinegar

5ml/1 tsp salt

1 Coarsely chop the preserved stem ginger. Slice the lime thinly, including the rind, then chop into small pieces. Place the cherry tomatoes, sugar, vinegar, salt, ginger and lime in a large heavy pan.

2 Bring to the boil, stirring until the sugar dissolves. Simmer rapidly for 45 minutes. Stir until the liquid has evaporated and the relish is thick and pulpy.

3 Leave to cool for about 5 minutes, then spoon into sterilized jars. Leave to cool, then cover and store in the refrigerator for up to 1 month.

Energy 530kcal/2262kJ; **Protein** 3.7g; **Carbohydrate** 134.1g, of which sugars 134.1g; **Fat** 1.4g, of which saturates 0.5g; **Cholesterol** 0mg; **Calcium** 93mg; **Fibre** 4.5g; **Sodium** 2012mg.

Cranberry and red onion relish

This sophisticated relish mixes the richness of caramelized onions with the tartness of cranberries and vinegar.

INGREDIENTS

Makes about 900g/2lb

30ml/2 tbsp olive oil

450g/1lb small red onions, finely sliced

225g/8oz/1 cup soft light brown sugar

450g/1lb/4 cups fresh or frozen cranberries

120ml/4fl oz/^{1}/2 cup red wine vinegar

120ml/4fl oz/^{1}/2 cup red wine

15ml/1 tbsp mustard seeds

2.5ml/^{1}/2 tsp ground ginger

30ml/2 tbsp orange liqueur or port

salt and ground black pepper

1 Heat the olive oil in a large pan, add the sliced onions and cook over a low heat for about 15 minutes, stirring occasionally, until they have softened.

2 Add 30ml/2 tbsp of the sugar and cook for a further 5 minutes, or until the onions are caramelized.

3 Meanwhile, put the cranberries in a pan with the remaining sugar, and the vinegar, wine, mustard seeds and ginger. Heat gently until the sugar has dissolved, then cover and bring to the boil. It is important to cover the pan when cooking the cranberries because they can pop out of the pan during cooking and are very hot.

4 Simmer for 15 minutes, until the berries have burst and are tender, then stir in the caramelized onions. Increase the heat slightly and cook uncovered for a further 10 minutes, stirring frequently until well reduced and thickened. Remove from the heat, then season to taste.

5 Transfer to warmed sterilized jars. Spoon a little of the orange liqueur or port over the top of each, then cover and seal. Store the jars in a cool place for up to 6 months. Once opened, store in the refrigerator and then use within 1 month.

Energy 1532kcal/6486kJ; **Protein** 8g; **Carbohydrate** 314.6g, of which sugars 304.2g; **Fat** 23.3g, of which saturates 3.2g; **Cholesterol** 0mg; **Calcium** 259mg; **Fibre** 13.5g; **Sodium** 46mg.

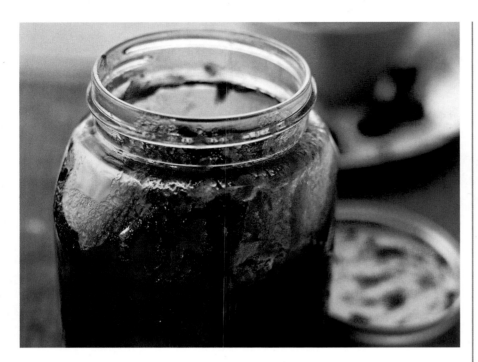

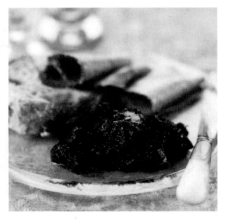

Kashmir chutney

This sweet, chunky, spicy chutney is perfect served with cold meats.

INGREDIENTS

Makes about 2.75kg/6lb

1kg/2^1/4lb green eating apples

15g/^{1}/2oz garlic cloves

1 litre/1^3/4 pints/4 cups malt vinegar

450g/1lb dates

115g/4oz preserved stem ginger

450g/1lb/3 cups raisins

450g/1lb/2 cups soft light brown sugar

2.5ml/^{1}/2 tsp cayenne pepper

30ml/2 tbsp salt

1 Quarter the apples, remove the cores and chop coarsely. Peel and chop the garlic.

2 Place the apple with the chopped garlic in a pan with enough vinegar to cover. Bring to the boil and boil for 10 minutes.

3 Chop the dates and ginger and add them to the pan, with the rest of the ingredients. Cook gently for 45 minutes.

4 Spoon the mixture into warmed sterilized jars and seal immediately. Store in a cool, dark place and use within 1 year. Once opened, store in the refrigerator and use within 2 months.

Energy 3920kcal/16,737kJ; **Protein** 22.6g; **Carbohydrate** 1014.4g, of which sugars 1012.2g; **Fat** 3.3g, of which saturates 0g; **Cholesterol** 0mg; **Calcium** 599mg; **Fibre** 33.7g; **Sodium** 12139mg.

Chunky pear and walnut chutney

The perfect balance of cider vinegar and tart apples and pears makes this a surprisingly mellow accompaniment to cheese as well as grains including pilaffs and tabbouleh.

INGREDIENTS

Makes about 1.8kg/4lb

1.2kg/2^1/2lb firm pears

225g/8oz tart cooking apples

225g/8oz onions

450ml/^{3}/4 pint/scant 2 cups cider vinegar

175g/6oz/generous 1 cup sultanas
  (golden raisins)

finely grated rind and juice of 1 orange

400g/14oz/2 cups sugar

115g/4oz/1 cup walnuts, roughly chopped

2.5ml/^{1}/2 tsp ground cinnamon

1 Peel and core the pears and apples, then chop them into 2.5cm/1in chunks. Peel and quarter the onions, then chop into pieces of the same size.

2 Place in a preserving pan with the vinegar. Slowly bring to the boil, then reduce the heat and simmer for 40 minutes, until the apples, pears and onions are tender, stirring occasionally.

3 Meanwhile, put the sultanas in a bowl, pour over the orange juice and leave to soak.

4 Add the sugar, sultanas, and orange rind and juice to the pan.

5 Gently heat the mixture until the sugar has dissolved, then simmer for 30–40 minutes, or until the chutney is thick and no excess liquid remains. Stir frequently towards the end of cooking to prevent the chutney sticking on the bottom of the pan.

6 Gently toast the walnuts in a non-stick pan over a low heat, stirring constantly, for 5 minutes, until golden. Stir the nuts into the chutney with the cinnamon.

7 Spoon the chutney into warmed sterilized jars, cover and seal. Store in a cool, dark place, then leave to mature for at least 1 month. Use within 1 year. Once opened, store in the refrigerator and use within 2 months.

Energy 3501kcal/14,797kJ; **Protein** 29.8g; **Carbohydrate** 705.3g, of which sugars 699.3g; **Fat** 81.4g, of which saturates 6.4g; **Cholesterol** 0mg; **Calcium** 603mg; **Fibre** 40.7g; **Sodium** 189mg.

VINEGAR IN JELLIES

Savoury jellies are classic accompaniments for roasted meats. Fruit or vegetables are cooked in vinegar and boiled with sugar to setting point.

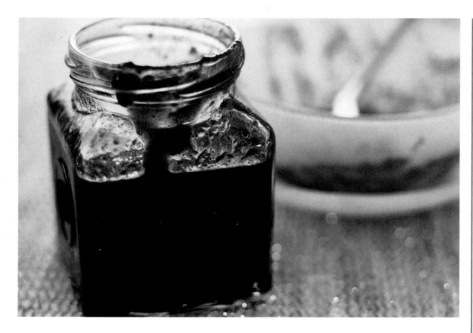

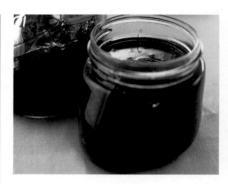

Plum and apple jelly

Serve this rich jelly with roast meats.

INGREDIENTS

Makes about 1.3kg/3lb

900g/2lb plums, stoned (pitted) and chopped

450g/1lb tart cooking apples, chopped

150ml/1/4 pint/2/3 cup cider vinegar

750ml/11/4 pints/3 cups water

675g/11/2lb/scant 31/2 cups sugar

1 In a pan, bring the fruit, vinegar and water to the boil, reduce the heat, cover and simmer for 30 minutes. Pour into a sterilized jelly bag suspended over a bowl.

2 Drain for 3 hours. Measure the juice into a pan, adding 450g/1lb/21/4 cups sugar for every 600ml/1 pint/21/2 cups juice. Bring to the boil, stirring, until the sugar dissolves. Boil for 10 minutes, or to setting point (105°C/220°F). Remove from heat and skim off scum. Pour into warmed sterilized jars. Cover and seal.

3 Store in a cool, dark place and use within 2 years. Once opened, keep refrigerated and use within 2 months.

Energy 2803kcal/11,963kJ; **Protein** 5.5g; **Carbohydrate** 740.7g, of which sugars 740.7g; **Fat** 0.4g, of which saturates 0g; **Cholesterol** 0mg; **Calcium** 401mg; **Fibre** 6.4g; **Sodium** 49mg.

Red pepper and chilli jelly

The hint of chilli in this jelly makes it ideal for spicing up sausages or burgers.

INGREDIENTS

Makes about 900g/2lb

8 red (bell) peppers, quartered and seeded

4 fresh red chillies, halved and seeded

1 onion, roughly chopped

2 garlic cloves, roughly chopped

250ml/8fl oz/1 cup water

250ml/8fl oz/1 cup white wine vinegar

7.5ml/11/2 tsp salt

450g/1lb/21/4 cups sugar

25ml/11/2 tbsp powdered pectin

1 Arrange the quartered red peppers, skin side up, on a rack in a grill (broiling) pan and grill (broil) until the skins blacken and blister.

2 Put the peppers in a polythene bag to steam for about 10 minutes, then carefully remove the skins.

3 Put the peppers, chillies, onion, garlic and water in a food processor and process to a purée. Press through a sieve (strainer) set over a bowl, pressing with a spoon to extract as much juice as possible. There should be about 750ml/11/4 pints/3 cups.

4 Scrape the purée into a large pan, then stir in the vinegar and salt. Combine the warmed sugar and pectin, then stir it into the puréed pepper mixture. Heat gently, stirring, until the sugar and pectin have dissolved, then bring to the boil.

5 Cook the jelly, stirring, for 4 minutes, then remove the pan from the heat. Pour into warmed, sterilized jars. Leave to cool and set, then cover, label and store in a cool dark place. Use within 1 year. Once opened, store in the refrigerator and use within 2 months.

Energy 2275kcal/9665kJ; **Protein** 18g; **Carbohydrate** 571g, of which sugars 565.1g; **Fat** 6.1g, of which saturates 1.5g; **Cholesterol** 0mg; **Calcium** 373mg; **Fibre** 24.8g; **Sodium** 89mg.

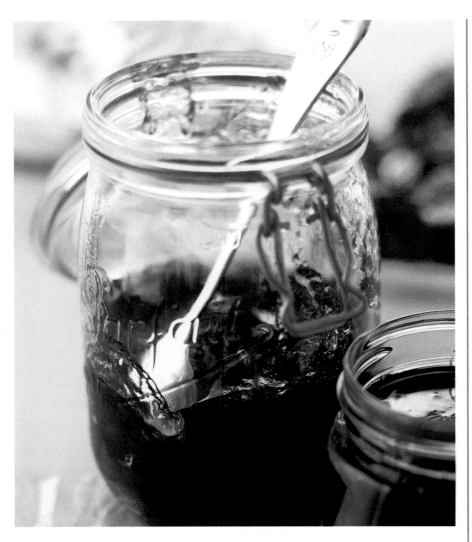

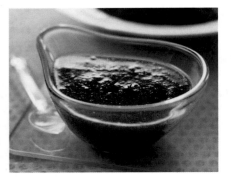

Tomato and herb jelly

This dark golden jelly is delicious served with grilled meats, especially lamb.

INGREDIENTS

Makes about 1.3kg/3lb

1.8kg/4lb tomatoes, washed and quartered

2 lemons, washed and chopped into pieces

2 bay leaves

250ml/**8** fl oz/1 cup malt vinegar

300ml/$^1/_2$ pint/1$^1/_4$ cups cold water

bunch of fresh rosemary

about 900g/2lb/4$^1/_2$ cups sugar

1 Put the tomatoes and lemons in a large pan with the bay leaves and add the vinegar and water. Add the rosemary, bring to the boil, then reduce the heat. Cover and simmer for 40 minutes, until the tomatoes are soft.

2 Pour into a sterilized jelly bag suspended over a bowl. Drain for 3 hours. Measure the juice into a clean pan, adding 450g/1lb/2$^1/_2$ cups juice. Heat gently, stirring, until the sugar dissolves. Boil for 10 minutes, to setting point (105°C/ 220°F), then remove from the heat. Skim off any scum. Leave for a few minutes until a skin forms.

3 Pour the jelly into sterilized jars. Cover and seal when cold. Store in a cool, dark place and use within 1 year. Once opened, keep chilled. Use within 3 months.

Energy 3767kcal/16078kJ; **Protein** 13.6g; **Carbohydrate** 980.8g, of which sugars 980.8g; **Fat** 3.9g, of which saturates 1.3g; **Cholesterol** 0mg; **Calcium** 568mg; **Fibre** 13g; **Sodium** 171mg.

Minted gooseberry jelly

This classic, tart jelly takes on a pinkish tinge during cooking, not green as one would expect.

INGREDIENTS

Makes about 1.2kg/2$^1/_2$lb

1.3kg/3lb/12 cups gooseberries

1 bunch fresh mint

750ml/1$^1/_4$ pints/3 cups cold water

400ml/14fl oz/1 $^2/_3$ cups white wine vinegar

about 900g/2lb/4$^1/_2$ cups preserving or granulated (white) sugar

45ml/3 tbsp chopped fresh mint

1 Place the gooseberries, mint and water in a preserving pan. Bring to the boil, reduce the heat, cover and simmer for 30 minutes, until the gooseberries are soft. Add the vinegar and simmer, uncovered, for a further 10 minutes.

2 Pour the fruit and juices into a sterilized jelly bag suspended over a bowl. Leave to drain for at least 3 hours, until the juices stop dripping, then measure the strained juices back into the cleaned preserving pan.

3 Add 450g/1lb/2$^1/_4$ cups sugar for every 600ml/1 pint/2$^1/_2$ cups juice, then heat gently, stirring, until dissolved. Bring to the boil. Cook for 15 minutes to setting point (105°C/220°F). Remove from the heat and skim off any scum. Cool until a thin skin forms, then stir in the mint.

4 Pour into sterilized jars, cover and seal. Use within 1 year. Once opened, keep chilled. Use within 3 months.

Energy 3641kcal/15,534kJ; **Protein** 10g; **Carbohydrate** 955.5g, of which sugars 955.5g; **Fat** 2g, of which saturates 0g; **Cholesterol** 0mg; **Calcium** 617mg; **Fibre** 12g; **Sodium** 64mg.

INDEX

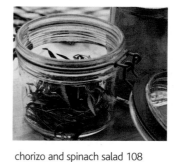

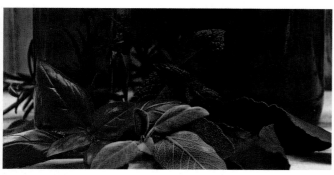

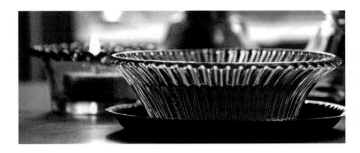

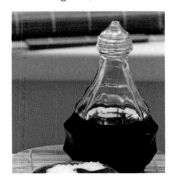

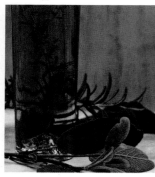

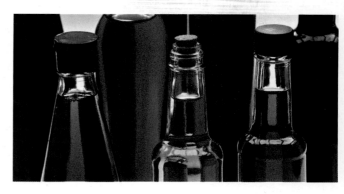

shoes
  odour prevention 61
shower fittings and curtains 75
sinus congestion 41, 44
skincare 11
  age spots 51
  blocked pores 40, 46
  chapped skin 46
  exfoliators 31, 40
  face packs see face packs
  face steaming 63
  oatmeal salt scrub 62
  oily skin 65
  open pores 65
  pH balance 54, 55, 56
  pore-opening 62, 63
  refreshing hot cloth 62
  rose petal toner 63
  rough skin scrub 60
  spots and blemishes 40
  stain removal 55, 58
  stimulating fruit paste 65
  vinegar 40–1, 46–7, 62–3
  vinegar, parsley and yogurt
    pack 65
  vinegar and rosewater
    freshener 63
  see also beauty products;
    footcare; haircare; handcare
skin complaints 38, 40
sloe vinegar 101
slug barrier, vinegar as 85
smoke, removing smell of 76
smoothies, vinegar 121
snails, edible 88
sore throats 41, 44
sorghum vinegar 23
sour cucumber with fresh dill
  111
spirit vinegar 28–9
spots and blemishes 40
sprayers, garden 85

spritzers, vinegar 119
stain removal
  carpets 73
  chopping boards 79
  cutlery 79
  from skin 55, 58
  furniture 70
  glass 79
  laundry 68
  mugs and cups 79
  textiles 68, 80, 81
stainless steel 68, 75, 78, 79
steak with warm tomato salsa
  115
stimulating fruit paste 65
stings and bites 40, 49, 85
stir-frying see frying
stone-fruit vinegar 101
storage
  pickles 15
  vinegar 10, 23
stoves, cleaning and polishing
  74
strawberry vinegar 101
stress 39, 42
su-meshi 32, 33
summer herb marinade 103
sunburn 41, 45
sushi rice 32, 33
sweet-sour/hot-sour flavours 11,
  29, 114
swimwear, cleaning 81
switchel 11

taps, cleaning 73
tarragon vinegar 98
tartare sauce 104
tartaric acid 14–15
tension 42
teriyaki marinade 103
textiles
  chewing gum, removal 72
  coloured 80, 81
  dishcloths 81
  removing shine 81
  rugs 72, 73
  scorched 80
  stain removal 68, 80, 81
  terry nappies 81
  yellowed fabric 80
thermos flasks, tainted 78
thyme
  marinade 103
  vinegar 98
tiles, cleaning 73
tins, cleaning 78
toilets, deodorizing 77
tomatoes
  steak with warm tomato salsa
    115
  tart tomato relish 122
  tomato and herb jelly 125
  tomato vinegar 34
toner, rose petal 63
tuna Niçoise, seared 112

vases, stained 79
vegetables
  discolouration 88, 95
Venetian blinds, cleaning 74

venison 88, 90
vinaigrette 102
vinegar
  acidity 8, 14–15
  as antibacterial 55
  as antiseptic 6, 9, 40, 41
  as astringent 6, 9, 40, 65
  beauty products 53–65
  as cleanser 9, 11, 15, 68–82
  culinary uses 88–125
  as disinfectant 40
  in drinks 120–1
  flavouring 96–7
  flowers, infused with 99
  food preparation 88
  four thieves vinegar 41
  grain 22, 23
  herbs, infused with 8, 68, 90,
    96, 98–9
  history of 8–9
  live 18–19
  macerating fruit 88, 91
  marinades 15, 88, 90–1, 103
  medicinal use see health and
    healing
  military uses 9
  nutritional value 38–9
  organic 22–3
  pasteurization 12
  as preservative 8, 11, 89,
    92–3
  in sauces 104–105
  scented 68
  seasoning with 8
  sherry 18, 22, 29
  spiced 8, 28, 29, 90, 93, 86–7
  storage 10, 23
  tasting 23
  as a tonic 38–9
  vegetable 23
  wine see wine vinegar
vinegar production 8, 12–13,
  24–5, 30
  history of 10–11
  making your own vinegar
    18–19, 30
  mother see mother of vinegar
  Orléans method 16, 26
  spiced vinegar 19
  wine vinegar 10
  yeasts 12–13
virgin prairie oyster 120

wallpaper, stripping 82
walnuts
  pear and walnut chutney 125

pickled 93
wasp stings 40, 49
waxy ear build-up 39
weed deterrent 85
weight loss 30, 31
wheat vinegar 23
whey vinegar 22
white vinegar 28–9, 54, 69, 74, 93
windows
  cleaning 68, 72, 84
  films, removal 72
windscreens and wipers, cleaning
  85
wine stains, removal 80
wine vinegar 10, 12–13, 18, 22,
  26–7
wood
  chopping boards 79
  cleaning and restoration 68,
    69
  mahogany bloom 70
  oil-based finishes 192
  polishing 193
  preservation 6
woodwork, preparation for paint
  82

yeasts 12–13

ACKNOWLEDGEMENTS AND PICTURE CREDITS

The author and publishers would like to thank the following companies for supplying vinegars: Aspall, Belazu, Blue Dragon, Clearspring, Delicious Fine Foods, Fieldhouse Farms, Hillfarm Oils, Meridian Foods, Suzanne's Vinegars.
Models: Kiera Blakey and Patrick Tubbritt.
Thanks to the following picture libraries for the use of their pictures in the book.
Alamy: 8b, 14, 17l, 18t, 24l, 24m, 25l, 35br, 40tr, 69bl, 84tr, 84br. **The Art Archive:** 10t. **Bridgeman Art Library:** 8t, 9t, 9b, 16. **Corbis:** 10b, 13b, 17m, 27l, 27m. **Getty Images:** 32m, 33tl, 35bl, 43t. **Istockphoto:** 72tr, 74br, 77tl, 77tr, 81tm, 81bm.

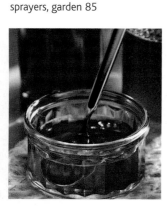